W0106238

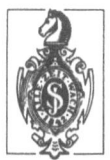

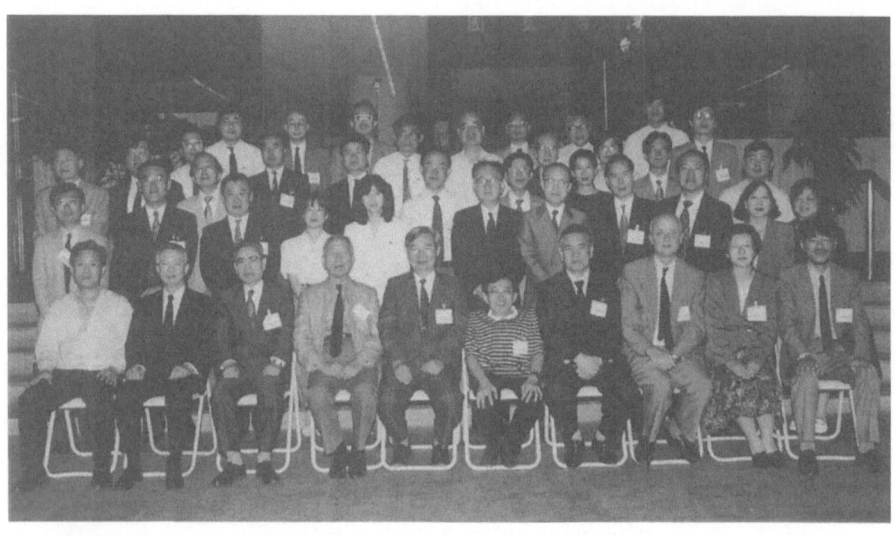

The Second Sino-Japanese Symposium on Coagulaton, Fibrinolysis, and Platelets,
October 3 - 5, 1992, Taipei, Taiwan.

M.-C. Shen · C.-M. Teng · A. Takada(Eds.)

Current Aspects of Blood Coagulation, Fibrinolysis, and Platelets

With 100 Figures

Springer Japan KK

MING-CHING SHEN
Professor and Chairman, Department of Laboratory Medicine, National Taiwan
University Hospital, Taipei, Taiwan

CHE-MING TENG
Professor and Chairman, Department of Pharmacology, College of Medicine, National
Taiwan University, Taipei, Taiwan

AKIKAZU TAKADA
Professor and Chairman, Department of Physiology, Hamamatsu University, School of
Medicine, Hamamatsu, Shizuoka, 431-31 Japan

ISBN 978-4-431-70123-1   ISBN 978-4-431-68323-0 (eBook)
DOI 10.1007/978-4-431-68323-0

Printed on acid-free paper

© Springer Japan 1993

Originally published by Springer-Verlag Tokyo Berlin Heidelberg New York in 1993

Preface

The first Sino-Japanese Symposium on Coagulation, Fibrinolysis and Platelets, originating from the Hamamatsu symposium, held in early 1990, was held in Hanchow, Mainland China in October, 1990. During that meeting, Taipei was selected as the next meeting place. We took great pleasure in carrying out this noble endeavor and were honored to have Professor Stenflo, Professor Hedner from Sweden, Professor Aoki and many other distinguished scientists from Japan joining us on this Second Sino-Japanese symposium. Our only regret was that our friends from Mainland China did not attend.

The topics covered during the 3-day symposium included areas of both basic and clinical research. The symposium has been an excellent opportunity for all the participants to exchange ideas and improve their expertise, and at the same time, to expand frontiers in the field of coagulation, fibrinolysis and platelets. The symposium was very successful both in terms of contributing greatly to raise the level of research and development in the field of thrombosis and hemostasis and in helping to promote international scientific cooperation and friendship.

We would like to express our appreciation to the members of our organizing and scientific committee for their devotion to this project. We also wish to thank our National Science Council and Department of Health, and the Asia and Pacific Council for Science and Technology, as well as the many other sponsors for their financial support. Without them, this instructive and invaluable symposium and this proceedings would not have been possible.

Oct. 6, 1992

Ming-Ching Shen
CHe-Ming Teng
Akikazu Takada

Taipei, R.O.C.

Contents

Coagulation and its regulation

Disorders of coagulation, fibrinolysis, platelets and thrombosis

Fibrinolysis

Platelets and antithrombotic agents

Coagulation and
its regulation

CALCIUM BINDING PROPERTIES OF VITAMIN K-DEPENDENT CLOTTING FACTORS.

J. STENFLO,[1] M. SELANDER[2] E. PERSSON,[1] J. ASTERMARK, [1] C. VALCARCE[1] AND T. DRAKENBERG.[2]

[1]Department of Clinical Chemistry, Lund University, Malmö General Hospital, S-214 01 Malmö, Sweden.
[2]Department of Physical Chemistry 2, Chemical Center, Lund University, POB 124, S-214 01 Lund, Sweden.

INTRODUCTION

Blood coagulation results form a series of activations of zymogens of serine proteases by limited proteolytic cleavage. These reactions form what is commonly referred to as a procoagulant cascade. The final zymogen activation is the conversion of prothrombin to thrombin, the latter subsequently cleaving four peptide bonds in soluble fibrinogen, which becomes transformed into insoluble fibrin (1-4). The procoagulant cascade is regulated by an anticoagulant counterpart, termed the "protein C anticoagulant system". An adequate balance between the pro- and anticoagulant systems is a prerequisite for the prevention of bleeding and/or thrombosis (5,6). The reactions in both pathways are carried out by macromolecular complexes (active enzyme and cofactor) assembled on the surface of phospholipid membranes, such as aggregated platelets or damaged cells. Assembly of these complexes requires that the zymogens and enzymes as well as the cofactors bind calcium. Calcium is thus crucial for blood coagulation to proceed normally. In this paper the calcium binding properties of vitamin K-dependent proteins involved in blood coagulation will be reviewed briefly.

The calcium requirement for blood coagulation was discovered more than 100 years ago. It was soon realized that calcium is not required for the conversion of fibrinogen to fibrin but in reaction(s) preceding this step (7). The identification of vitamin K in the 1930s and the demonstration that it is required for normal biosynthesis of certain coagulation factors was an important step forward, as was the identification of the vitamin K antagonist dicoumarol and the chemical synthesis of active dicoumarol analogues, such as warfarin (8,9). In the 1950s and 60s it was found that phospholipid surfaces enhance the rate of, for instance, prothrombin activation to thrombin and that the interaction between prothrombin and phospholipid surfaces is calcium-dependent (7). Vitamin K function was linked to calcium binding when it was demonstrated that patients treated with a vitamin K antagonists, such as dicoumarol or warfarin, synthesized abnormal forms of prothrombin which appeared not to bind calcium (10). This observation made possible the identification in 1974 of γ-carboxyglutamic acid (Gla) as the vitamin K-dependent structure first in prothrombin, and then in factors VII, IX, X, protein C, and protein S (10-13).

It is now well established that the vitamin K-dependent clotting factors are composed of multiple domains or modules (in the following the term module will be used (14,15)), most of which are encoded on separate exons (12,14). The calcium-binding Gla module is N-terminal in all these proteins. In prothrombin it is followed by two kringle modules and in factors VII, IX, X and protein C by two modules homologous to the epidermal growth factor (EGF). The serine protease module occupies the C-terminal half of each protein. The structure of factor X is illustrated schematically in Fig. 1. In protein S, a cofactor to activated protein C, the Gla module is followed by a thrombin-sensitive module and four EGF-like modules, whereas the C-terminal part of the molecule is homologous to a steroid hormone-binding plasma protein (16,17). The structure of the proteins suggested that proteolytic cleavage between modules was possible, which would allow subsequent isolation of intact modules. With this approach it became possible to investigate whether calcium binding is confined to the Gla module or whether other modules also bind calcium. The first step along this line was the removal of the Gla module by limited

4

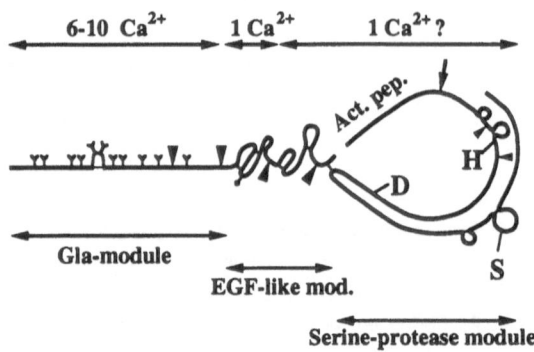

Fig. 1. *Schematic diagram of the structure of factor X showing the location of calcium-binding sites. The arrow denotes where cleavage occurs during activation ov factor X and the arrowheads denote the loacations of introns.*

chymotryptic cleavage, first from factor X and then from protein C (18,19). Studies of calcium binding to protein C lacking the Gla module established the presence of functionally important Gla-independent calcium binding site(s) in this protein (19,20).

Gla-CONTAINING MODULES. STRUCTURE AND CALCIUM BINDING PROPERTIES.

Each vitamin K-dependent plasma protein contains an N-terminal, approximately 47-amino-acids long module with 10-12 Gla residues formed by postribosomal carboxylation of Glu. In vitamin K deficiency or during treatment with vitamin K-antagonistic drugs, hepatic carboxylation of the appropriate Glu residues is inhibited and uncarboxylated or partially carboxylated proteins are secreted (10-13). A propeptide, removed by limited proteolysis prior to secretion, is the structure recognized by the vitamin K-dependent carboxylase (12, 13,21). The propeptide and the N-terminal 37 or 38 residues of the mature protein are encoded on the same exon, whereas the following 8 residues, which form an α-helix with a cluster of aromatic amino acids, are encoded on a separate exon (2,22). In factors IX and X the α-helical region contains one Gla residue. The types of splice junctions at intron-exon boundaries support the notion that the propeptide-Gla region is a functional unit that has been subjected to gene duplication, point mutations and exon shuffling (14).

The carboxylation of Glu residues leads to an increased calcium affinity. This is illustrated by the fact that a monocarboxylic acid such as acetic acid binds calcium with a K_d of approximately 300 mM, whereas malonic acid, a dicarboxylic acid, similar to the sidechain of Gla, binds calcium with higher affinity, K_d of approximately 30 mM, though, still far above the calcium concentration in plasma (23). The vitamin K-dependent proteins have 8-12 calcium binding sites. Two or three of these sites bind calcium with positive cooperativity (23-26). This characteristic cooperative binding presupposes a native conformation in the Gla module, e.g. upon reduction and alkylation of the single disulfide bond in the Gla module the cooperative calcium binding is lost. Moreover, in the absence of calcium the structure of the Gla module appears to be disordered, as judged by X-ray crystallography. The vitamin K-dependent proteins also bind divalent cations, such as Mn^{2+}, Mg^{2+} and Sr^{2+}. Although binding of these ions mimics some of the alterations in properties induced by calcium, such as quenching of the intrinsic Trp fluorescence, they can not substitute for calcium in blood coagulation (23).

Recently, the three-dimensional structure of bovine prothrombin fragment 1, which consists of the Gla module, a tetradecapeptide disulfide loop and the first kringle module, was determined by X-ray crystallography. In the absence of calcium the structure of the N-terminal 35 residues of the Gla module was disordered, except for the disulfide bond connecting Cys 18 and 23, whereas the C-terminal a-helix was ordered (27). In the presence of calcium, however, the Gla module was found to have the shape of a discoid and a well defined structure, that has now been solved to 2.2 Å resolution (22,28). The main features of the structure are as follows: The α-helix that is C-terminal in the Gla module, residues 38 to 46, contains a cluster of aromatic amino acids (Phe 41, Trp 42 and Tyr 45). This part, which is ordered also in the absence of calcium, is presumably a nucleation site in the calcium-induced folding of the N-terminal part of the Gla module. It is separated by a short stretch of peptide form two turns of α-helix (residues 25 to 31; Fig. 2). This region is followed by the hexapeptide disulfide loop connecting Cys 18 and 23, which is adjacent to the aromatic cluster in the α-helix, and a single turn of α-helix (residues 14 to 17). The N-terminal residues are folded in a loop resembling the letter Ω with the N-terminus buried and making an ion pair interaction with either of Gla 17, 21 or 27.

The three-dimensional structure of the calcium form of the Gla module demonstrates that the metal ions interact with carboxylate groups of Gla residues which are remote in the linear sequence and thus seem to crosslink different parts of the module. It is noteworthy that Gla residues 17, 26, 27 and 30 form a negatively charged surface, apposing the carboxylate groups of Gla residues 7 and 8. Four to five calcium ions are interposed between the negatively charged surfaces. Gla residues 15, 20 and 21 seem to form a loose calcium cluster which is exposed to solvent. Moreover, Gla 15 forms an ion pair with Arg 55 in the tetradecapeptide loop, suggesting that this region supports folding of the Gla module. The negatively charged surfaces formed by Gla sidechains explain the cooperative calcium ion binding.

The pronounced sequence similarity suggests that the Gla modules of all vitamin K-dependent coagulation factors are folded in essentially the same manner (2). This notion is also supported by the results of chemical modification experiments (29), as well as those of experiments using crossreacting monoclonal antibodies (30) and, most important, similar calcium binding properties (23). For instance, the intrinsic protein fluorescence is quenched upon calcium binding to the Gla modules of all the vitamin K-dependent clotting factors (31-35), presumably due to interaction between the disulfide bond between Cys 18 and 23 and the indole of Trp 42 in the aromatic cluster (28).

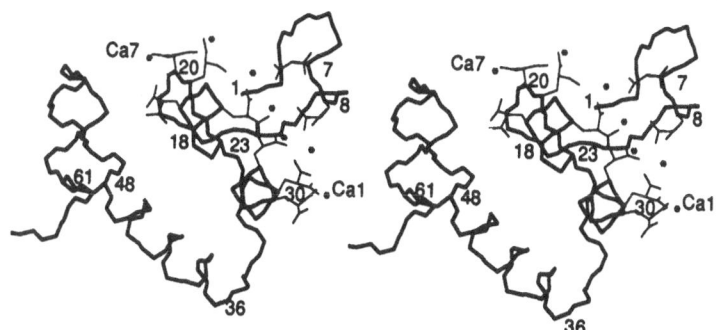

Fig. 2. Stereoview of the structure of the Gla module in bovine prothrombin fagment 1. The polypeptide backbone and the side chains of the Gla residues are shown. The filled circles denote calcium ions. Reproduced with permission from M. Soriano-Garcia and coworkers (28).

Binding of calcium to the Gla residues is a prerequisite for normal interaction of the vitamin K-dependent clotting factors with negatively charged (phosphatidyl serine-containing) phospholipid surfaces and biological activity (10,11). Accordingly, the uncarboxylated or partially carboxylated clotting factors synthesized during treatment with vitamin K antagonists, which have Glu instead of Gla, do not bind calcium and do not interact with biological membranes. The role of the phospholipid membranes is illustrated by the activation of prothrombin by active factor X (factor Xa). Addition of phospholipid vesicles (e.g. single compartment phospholipid vesicles containing 75 % phosphatidyl choline and 25 % phosphatidyl serine) to a reaction mixture containing factor Xa, prothrombin and calcium results in a lowering of the K_m for prothrombin by more than two orders of magnitude (3). This effect is not obtained with the corresponding uncarboxylated proteins. Already the loss of three or four Gla residues results in a marked reduction in phospholipid binding and biological activity (36). From the three-dimensional structure of the Gla modules it is obvious that the Gla residues are not functionally equivalent. This is also illustrated by findings in studies of mutant factors IX, X and protein C with point mutations affecting Gla residues. All these mutant proteins have low biological activity but the severity of the defect varies depending on which residue is mutated (37-40).

The interaction between the Gla-containing coagulation factors and biological membranes have long been thought to be ionic in nature, with calcium ions mediating the interaction between the Gla residues and the negatively charged phospholipid surface. This model must now be revised in the light of the three-dimensional structure of the Gla module of prothrombin fragment 1 (28). For instance, only few of the Gla residues are exposed on the surface of the module and available for participation in a calcium ion-mediated interaction with the phospholipid surface. At this stage, the present structure of prothrombin fragment 1 does not provide an immediately obvious answer to the question how the Gla module mediates the interaction with phospholipid surfaces. However, the structure provides a firm foundation for future studies aimed at elucidating this question, for instance by means of site-directed mutagenesis.

Normal vitamin K-dependent carboxylation of the Gla modules is required not only for calcium binding and normal interaction with phospholipid membranes, but also for normal transport of the protein through the endoplasmatic reticulum of the hepatocytes to the blood plasma (10,11). Accordingly, patients treated with vitamin K antagonistic drugs such as warfarin typically have a prothrombin concentration in blood plasma that is approximately 50 % of normal, though, the *biological activity* of prothrombin and the vitamin K-dependent proteins is much lower due to the defective carboxylation (41). Moreover, the Gla residues appear to be required for normal interaction of protein C with the cofactor thrombomodulin and for the interaction of factor VIIa with its cofactor, tissue factor (42,43).

THE EPIDERMAL GROWTH FACTOR-LIKE MODULES. STRUCTURE AND CALCIUM BINDING PROPERTIES.

Modules homologous to the epidermal growth factor (EGF) have been found in numerous extracellular and membrane proteins. They have a characteristic pattern of three disulfide bonds with the Cys residues linked 1-3, 2-4 and 5-6 (44-47). Among the vitamin K-dependent proteins, factors VII, IX, X and protein C each have two such modules located between the Gla module and the C-terminal serine protease part, whereas protein S, the vitamin K-dependent cofactor to protein C, has four such modules. The first EGF-like module in factors IX, X, protein C and protein S has one hydroxylated Asp residue, *erythro*-β-hydroxyaspartic acid (Hya), in a characteristic position (Fig. 3). In protein S, EGF-like domains 2-4 have one *erythro*-β-hydroxyasparagin (Hyn) residue each (47). The two modified amino acids formed by postribosomal hydroxylation of Asp and Asn respectively appear to be hydroxylated by the same enzyme, an Asp/Asn-β-hydroxylase (48). The enzyme is an α-ketoglutarate-dependent dioxygenase, related to prolyl-4-hydroxylase (49,50). Hydroxylation requires the consensus Cys-Xxx-Asp[*]/Asn[*]-Xxx-Xxx-Xxx-Xxx-Tyr/Phe-Xxx-Cys, corresponding to residues 61 to 70 in factor X (51,52). The asterisks denote the hydroxylated residue.

Recently, the structures of the N-terminal EGF-like modules in factors IX and X have been determined by 2D NMR methods and simulated folding (53-55). The fold was found to be similar to those of EGF and TGF-α. The structures are dominated by β-sheets and β-turns. In factor X there is a major β-sheet encompassing residues 59 to 63 and 68 to 72 whereas there are turns and shorter β-sheets in the C-terminal half of the module. Note that the Hya residue (denoted by β in Fig. 3) is adjacent to the conserved Tyr/Phe residue in the major β-sheet. In contrast to EGF, however, the residues N-terminal of the first Cys in factors IX and X do not line up with the major β-sheet (55,56).

The Hya-containing EGF-like modules of factors IX, X and protein C bind one calcium ion with moderate affinity (57-59). Binding of calcium to this site has been studied both in the isolated EGF-like modules and in proteolytic fragments consisting of the Gla module linked to the N-terminal EGF-like module, e.g. fX-GlaEGF$_N$(34, 35, 55, 58, 59). Binding of calcium to fX-GlaEGF$_N$ and similar fragments is accompanied by an initial increase in the intrinsic tryptophan fluorescence due to metal binding to the site in the EGF-like module. At higher calcium concentrations there is a pronounced fluorescence quenching caused by calcium binding to sites in the Gla module. Accordingly, calcium titrations of fX-GlaEGF$_N$, after decarboxylation of the Gla residues by heat treatment, result in the characteristic fluorescence increase caused by calcium binding to the site in the EGF-like module, whereas the fluorescence quenching characteristic of binding to the Gla residues is absent (34). NMR spectroscopy can be used to monitor the binding of calcium both to fX-EGF$_N$ and fX-GlaEGF$_N$, as calcium binding alters the chemical shift of a well resolved signal, associated with the Tyr residue that is adjacent to the Hya in the major pleated sheet (54,55,58). These studies have established that fX-EGF$_N$ binds calcium with a K_d of approximately 700 μM. However, when the EGF and Gla modules are linked the affinity of the site in the EGF-like module is characterized by a K_d of approximately 70 μM, suggesting residue(s) in the Gla module to be involved in the metal ion binding (unpublished result). Moreover, the site in the EGF-like module is almost saturated before calcium binds to sites in the Gla module (unpublished result).

Early studies of the calcium binding to factors IX, X and protein C, from which the Gla modules have been removed by limited proteolytic cleavage in the aromatic stack region of the Gla modules, yielded one or two sites with K_d values ranging from 40 to 200 μM as estimated with equilibrium dialysis (19,20). In this context it is noteworthy that the affinity of the calcium binding site in the N-terminal EGF-like module of factor X is reduced approximately 10-fold when the Gla module is removed by proteolytic cleavage in the aromatic stack region (unpublished result). The contribution of the site in the N-terminal EGF-like module in factors IX and X and protein C to the calcium binding of the Gla-domainless proteins may thus be variable and, owing to the low affinity, difficult to measure accurately, particularly with equilibrium dialysis.

Based on the solution structure of EGF itself, it has been hypothesized that residues in factor IX that correspond to the two conserved Asp residues in positions 46 and 48 and the Hya residue in position 63 in factor X are calcium ligands (56). In factor IX, mutation of these residues results in the biosynthesis of factor IX with low biological activity (60). Moreover, the corresponding synthetic EGF-like modules have a greatly reduced calcium affinity (61). Finally, patients with hemophilia B have been identified where the mutant factor IX molecules have the residues implicated in calcium binding mutated (corresponding to positions 46, 49, and 63 in factor X; Fig. 3). These mutant factor IX molecules have low biological activity, and in one instance defective calcium binding has been demonstrated (62).

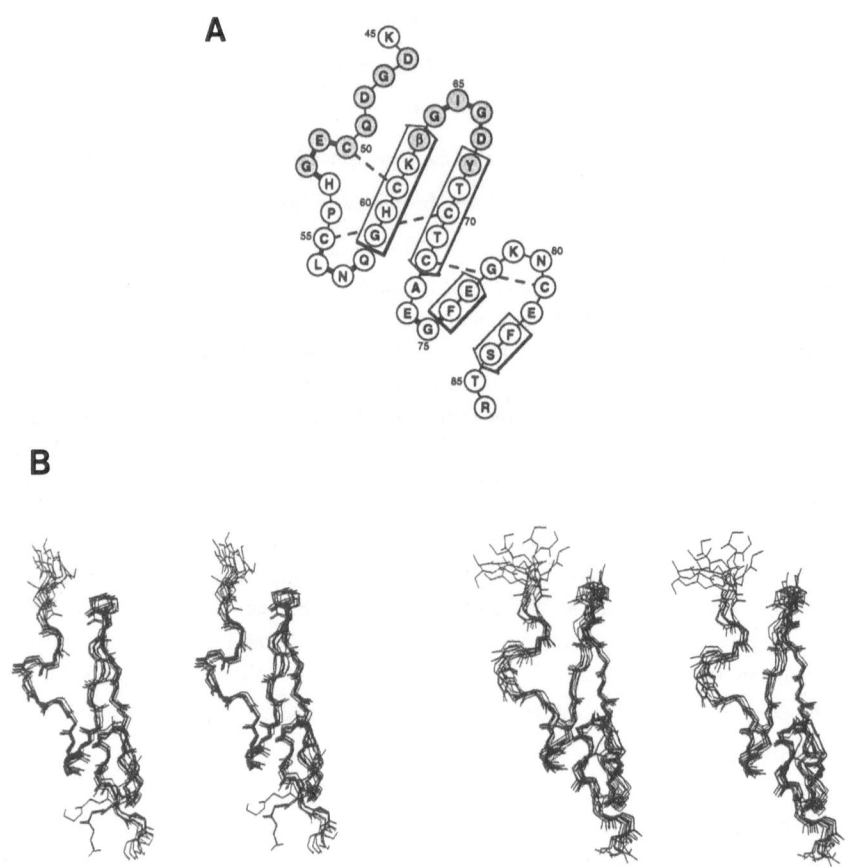

Fig. 3. A: Schematic diagram illustrating secondary structure features of the N-terminal EGF-like module in bovine factor X. Amino acids involved in calcium-binding are shaded. B: Stick representation in stereo in the same orientation of the calcium loaded (Left) and apo (Right) forms of the N-terminal EGF-like module from factor X. Structures were determined by 2D NMR and simulated folding. Reproduced with permission from Selander, M. and coworkers (55).

The structure of the EGF-like module from factor X has now been determined in the presence of calcium (55). The single calcium ion influences the structure of the N-terminal residues and the major β-sheet but does not alter the global fold of the module (Fig. 3). The calcium binding results in a better defined structure in this region with the N-terminal residues fixed on top of the major β-sheet. A shallow groove of a size appropriate to accomodate a calcium ion is formed. Five ligands to the calcium ion have been identified: the backbone carbonyls of Gly 47 and Gly 64; the sidechain carbonyl of Gln 49; the carboxyl of Hya 63; and, probably, the sidechain carboxyl of Asp 46. Calcium ions often have seven ligands and the final ligands in this site may be water molecules or ligands from the Gla module (63). It is noteworthy that Asp 48 appears not to be a calcium ligand. Nevertheless the negative charge of the sidechain carboxyl can contribute to the affinity of the site.

It should also be born in mind that the above studies have shed no light on the function of the hydroxyl group in the Hya residue. On calcium binding to the site, the β-COOH and -OH groups are rotated 120° around the α-β carbon axis such that in the calcium liganded form the -OH group faces away from the calcium ion (55). It is possible that in the intact protein the -OH group in the calcium liganded form may be hydrogen bonded to another part of the molecule or may interact with another protein. However, so far no calcium-dependent protein-protein interaction has been identified which involves the N-terminal EGF-like module in any of these proteins. The molecular mechanisms underlying the defective clotting associated with point mutations affecting those residues in the N-terminal EGF-like module that are calcium ligands thus remain to be elucidated.

In protein S, which has four EGF-like modules, the N-terminal one contains Hya and the three following ones Hyn (52). There are four high affinity Gla-independent calcium binding sites in protein S with calcium affinities ranging from 10 nM to 1 mM, at least two of which are located in the EGF-like modules (64). The functions of these modules and the calcium binding sites have not yet been elucidated. It should be noted, however, that the calcium affinity of the sites in the EGF-like modules in protein S are two to three orders of magnitude higher than the affinity of the corresponding sites in factors IX, X and protein C (47). This may be related to the fact that, whereas the latter factors have the consensus Asp-Gly-Asp-Gln-Cys corresponding to residues 46-50 in factor X, two of the protein S modules, which have Hyn instead of Hya, have the sequence Asp-Ile/Val-Asp-Glu-Cys. The substitution of Ile/Val for Gly and of Glu for Gln in all likelihood increases the calcium affinity of the site. In this context it should be noted that numerous non-vitamin K-dependent proteins contain the Asp-Ile/Val-Asp-Glu-Cys consensus as well as the consensus required by the Asp/Asn-β-hydroxylase (45,47,55). A few of these proteins have now been found to contain hydroxylated Asp/Asn in the position predicted by the consensus (47, 51, 65). Preliminary evidence suggests that some of these proteins bind calcium (66). Among these proteins are thrombomodulin, the EGF precursor, the gene products of the Notch and Delta loci in *Drosophila melanogaster* and fibrillin, the protein implicated in Marfan syndrome (47,67,68). It now appears safe to predict that many of the EGF-like modules in these proteins bind calcium, whether the appropriate Asp/Asn residues are hydroxylated or not.

CALCIUM BINDING SITES IN SERINE PROTEASE MODULES

When the three-dimensional structure of trypsin was determined by X-ray crystallography a single calcium binding site was identified (69,70). The bound calcium ion seems to inhibit the degradation of trypsin by autocatalysis. It is complexed by six ligands; a single water molecule, the sidechain carboxyl groups of Glu 52 and 62 (the numbering begins with the first residue in the active enzyme; Fig. 4), the backbone carbonyls of Asn 54 and Val 57, and finally the sidechain of Glu 59 by means of a hydrogen-bonded water molecule (70). These residues form a surface loop on the trypsin molecule.

In thrombin, which does not bind calcium, the two Glu residues, that are calcium ligands in trypsin, have been replaced by Lys and Ile, respectively (Fig. 4). However, in factors VII, IX, X and protein C the negative charge has been conserved in the corresponding positions. Recently, evidence was presented which indicated that factor IX has a calcium binding site in this region with a K_d of approximately 500 μM (71). Note that the three Glu residues that are sidechain ligands in trypsin are conserved in factor IX.

It is not yet known whether this calcium binding site is also present in factors VII, X and protein C. Preliminary evidence suggests that the corresponding region in factors IXa and Xa interact with the cofactors, factors VIIIa and Va, respectively (72,73).

The functional significance of Gla-independent calcium binding sites was first identified in protein C (19,20). Activation of protein C, from which the Gla module had been removed by limited proteolysis, was found to be calcium-dependent. The rate of activation of protein C lacking the Gla module with thrombin alone was inhibited by calcium, whereas the rate of activation with thrombin-thrombomodulin increased. These effects were attributed to a calcium binding site with a K_d of approximately 40 μM (19). Calcium binding to the modified protein resulted in a quenching of the intrinsic protein fluorescence. Recently, a deletion mutant of protein C, which lacks the Gla module and the N-terminal EGF-like module, was expressed (74). The calcium dependence of the activation of the mutant was identical with that of protein C lacking the Gla module. Moreover, the calcium-induced quenching of the intrinsic protein fluorescence was identical in the deletion mutant and in protein C lacking the Gla module. These results rule out the possibility that the calcium-binding site in the N-terminal EGF-like module is important for the activation of protein C lacking the Gla module. It remains to be elucidated whether protein C has a calcium-binding site in the serine protease part, similar to that in trypsin, and whether such a putative site explains the effects of calcium on the activation of protein C lacking the Gla module.

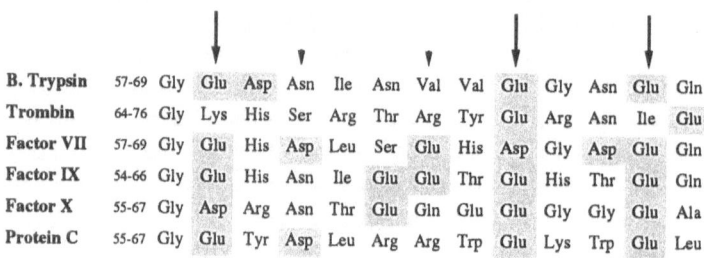

Fig. 4. Amino acid sequence in the calcium-binding region of bovine trypsin and the corresponding regions of vitamin K-dependent serine proteases. Among the latter proteins a calcium-binding site has so far only been found in factor IX. Glu and Asp residues are shaded. Residues with backbone carbonyl oxygens that are calcium ligands in trypsin are denoted with arrowheads and residues sidechain carboxyl groups that are calcium ligands are denoted with arrows. Amino acids are numbered beginning with the residue that is N-terminal in the serine protease module after activation.

REFERENCES

1. Jackson, C. M. and Nemerson, Y. (1980) *Ann Rev Biochem* **49**, 765-81.1

2. Furie, B. and Furie, B. C. (1988) *Cell* **53**, 505-518.

3. Mann, K. G., Nesheim, M. E., Church, W. R., Haley, P., and Krishnaswamy, S. (1990) *Blood.* **76**, 1-16.

4. Davie, E. W., Fujikawa, K., and Kisiel, W. (1991) *Biochemistry* **30**, 10363-10370.

5. Esmon, C. T. (1989) *J. Biol. Chem.* **264**, 4743-4746.

6. Stenflo, J. (1988) in *Protein C and Related Proteins* , (Bertina, R. M., ed) Churchill Livingstone, pp. 21-54.

7. Suttie, J. W. and Jackson, C. M. (1977) *Physiol. Rev.* **57**, 1-70.

8. Dam, H. (1935) *Biochem. J.* **29**, 1273-1285.

9. Campbell, H. A. and Link, K. P. (1941) *J. Biol. Chem.* **138**, 21-33.

10. Stenflo, J. and Suttie, J. W. (1977) *Ann. Rev. Biochem.* **46**, 157-172.

11. Suttie, J. (1985) *Ann. Rev. Biochem.* **54**, 459-477.

12. Furie, B. and Furie, B. C. (1990) *Blood.* **75**, 1753-1762.

13. Vermeer, C. (1990) *Biochem. J.* **266**, 625-636.

14. Patthy, L. (1985) *Cell* **41**, 657-663.

15. Baron, M., Norman, D. G., and Campbell, I. D. (1991) *Trends in Biochemical Sciences* **16**, 13-17.

16. Dahlbäck, B., Lundwall, Å., and Stenflo, J. (1986) *J. Biol. Chem.* **261**, 5111-5115.

17. Gershagen, S., Fernlund, P., and Lundwall, Å. (1987) *FEBS Lett.* **220**, 129-135.

18. Morita, T. and Jackson, C. . M. (1986) *J. Biol. Chem.* **261**, 4015-4023.

19. Esmon, N. L., DeBault, L. E., and Esmon, C. T. (1983) *J. Biol. Chem.* **258**, 5548-5553.

20. Johnson, A. E., Esmon, N. L., Laue, T. M., and Esmon, C. T. (1983) *J. Biol. Chem.* **258**, 5554-5560.

21. Hubbard, B, R., Jacobs, M., Ulrich, M. M. W., Furie, B. and Furie, B. C. (1990) *J. Biol. Chem.* **264**, 14145-14150.

22. Soriano-Garcia, M., Park, C. H., Tulinsky, A., Ravichandran, K. G., and Skrzypczak-Jankun, E. (1989) *Biochemistry* **28**, 6805-6810.

23. Jackson, C. M. (1988) in *Current Advances in Vitamin K Research*, (Suttie, J. W., ed) New York, Elsevier, pp. 305-324.

24. Stenflo, J. and Ganrot, P. (1974) *Biochem. Biophys. Res. Commun.* **50**, 98-104.

25. Bajaj, S. P., Butkowski, R. L., and Mann, K. G. (1975) *J. Biol. Chem.* **250**, 2150-2156.

26. Henriksen, R. A. and Jackson, C. M. (1975) *Arch. Biochem. Biophys.* **170**, 149-159.

27. Skrzypczak Jankun, E., Carperos, V. E., Ravichandran, K. G., and Tulinsky, A. (1992) *J. Mol. Biol.* **221**, 1379-1391.

28. Soriano-Garcia, M., Padmanabhan, K., deVos, A. M., and Tulinsky, A. (1992) *Biochemistry* **31**, 2554-2566.

29. Welsch, D. J., Pletcher, C. H., and Nelsestuen, G. L. (1988) *Biochemistry.* **27**, 4933-4938.

30. Church, W. R., Boulanger, L. L., Messier, T. L., and Mann, K. G. (1989) *J. Biol. Chem.* **264**, 17882-17887.

31. Nelsestuen, G. L. (1976) *J. Biol. Chem.* **25**, 5648-5656.

32. Prendergast, F. . G. and Mann, K. G. (1977) *J. Biol. Chem.* **252**, 840-850.

33. Öhlin, A. K., Björk, I., and Stenflo, J. (1990) *Biochemistry* **29**, 644-651.

34. Persson, E., Björk, I. and Stenflo, J. (1991) *J. Biol. Chem.*. **266**, 2444-2452.

35. Astermark, J., Björk, I., Öhlin, A-K. and Stenflo, J. (1991) *J. Biol. Chem.* **266**, 2430-2437.

36. Malhotra, O. P., Nesheim, M. E., and Mann, K. G. (1985) *J. Biol. Chem.* **260**, 279-287.

37. Gianelli, F., Green, P. M., High, K. A., Sommer, S., Lillicrap, D. P., Ludwig, M., Olek, K., Reitsma, P. H., Gossens, M., Yoshioka, A., and Brownlee, G. G. (1991) *Nucleic Acids Research* **19**, 2193-2219.

38. Watzke, H. H., Lechner, K., Roberts, H. R., Reddy, S. V., Welch, D. J., Friedman, P., Mahr, G., Jagadeeswaran, P., Monroe, D. M., and High, K. A. (1990) *J. Biol. Chem.* **265**, 11982-11989.

39. Zhang, L. and Castellino, F. J. (1990) *Biochemistry* **29**, 19828-19834.

40. Zhang, L. and Castellino, F. J. (1991) *Biochemistry* **30**, 6696-6704.

41. Ganrot, P. O. and Niléhn, J. E. (1968) *Scand. J. Clin. Lab. Invest.* **22**, 23-28.

42. Sakai, T., Lund Hansen, T., Thim, L., and Kisiel, W. (1990) *J. Biol. Chem.* **265**, 1890-1894.

43. Hogg, P. J., Öhlin, A-K., and Stenflo, J. (1992) *J. Biol. Chem.* **267**, 703-706.

44. Carpenter, G. and Cohen, S. (1990) *J. Biol. Chem.* **265**, 7709-7712.

45. Appella, E., Weber, I. T., and Blasi, F. (1988) *FEBS Lett.* **231**, 1-4.

46. Engel, J. (1989) *FEBS Lett.* **251**, 1-7.

47. Stenflo, J. (1991) *Blood* **78**, 1637-1651.

48. Wang, Q., VanDusen, W. J., Petroski, C. J., Garsky, V. M., Stern, A. M., and Friedman, P. A. (1991) J. Biol. Chem. **266**, 14004-14010.

49. Stenflo, J., Holme, E., Lindstedt, S., Chandramouli, N., Tsai Huang, L. H., Tam, J., and Merrifield, R. B. (1989) *Proc. Natl. Acad. Sci. USA* **86**, 444-447.

50. Gronke, R. S., VanDusen, W. J., Garsky, V. M., Jacobs, J. W., Saranda, . M. K., Stern, A. M., and Friedman, P. A. (1989) *Proc. Natl. Acad. Sci. USA* **86**, 3609-3613.

51. Stenflo, J., Öhlin, A. K., Owen, W. G., and Schneider, W. J. (1988) *J. Biol. Chem.* **263**, 21-24.

52. Stenflo, J., Lundwall, Å., and Dahlbäck, B. (1987) *Proc. Natl. Acad. Sci. USA* **84**, 368-372.

53. Baron, M., Norman, D. G., Harvey, T. S., Handford, P. A., Mayhew, M., Tse, A. G. D., Brownlee, G. G., and Campbell, I. D. (1992) *Protein Science* **1**, 81-90.

54. Ullner, M., Selander, M., Persson, E., Stenflo, J., Teleman, O., and Drakenberg, T. (1992) *Biochemistry* **31**, 5974-5983.

55. Selander, M., Ullner, M., Persson, E., Teleman, O., Stenflo, J., and Drakenberg, T. (1992) *J. Biol. Chem.* **267**, 19642-19649.

56. Cooke, R. M., Wilkinson, A. J., Baron, M., Pastore, A., Tappin, M. J., Campbell, I. D., Gregory, H., and Sheard, B. (1987) *Nature* **327**, 339-341.

57. Handford, P. A., Baron, M., Mayhew, M., Wills, A., Beesley, T., Brownlee, G. G., and Campbell, I. D. (1990) *EMBO J.* **9**, 475-480.

58. Persson, E., Selander, . M., Linse, S., Drakenberg, T., Öhlin, A.-K., and Stenflo, J. (1989) *J. Biol. Chem.* **264**, 16897-16904.

59. Öhlin, A. K., Linse, S., and Stenflo, J. (1988) *J. Biol. Chem.* **263**, 7411-7417.

60. Rees, D. J. G., Jones, I. M., Handford, P. A., Walter, S. J., Esnouf, M. P., Smith, K. J., and Brownlee, G. G. (1988) *EMBO J.* **7**, 2053-2061.

61. Handford, P. A., Mayhew, M., Baron, M., Winship, P. R., Campbell, I. D., and Brownlee, G. G. (1991) *Nature* **351**, 164-167.

62. McCord, D. M., Monroe, D. M., Smith, K. J., and Roberts, H. R. (1990) *J. Biol. Chem.* **265**, 10250-10254.

63. Strynadka, N. C. J. and James, M. N. G. (1991) *Current Opinion in Structural Biology* **1**, 905-914.

64. Dahlbäck, B., Hildebrand, B., and Linse, S. (1990) *J. Biol. Chem.* **265**, 18481-18489.

65. Kanazaki, T., Olofsson, A., Morén, A., Wernstedt, C., Hellman, U., Miyazono, K., Claesson Welsh, L., and Heldin, C. H. (1990) *Cell* **61**, 1051-1061.

66. Fehon, R. G., Kooh, P. J., Rebay, I., Regan, C. L., Xu, T., Muskavitch, M. A. T., and Artavanis Tsakonas, S. (1990) *Cell* **61**, 523-534.

67. Lee, B., Godfrey, M., Vitale, E., Hori, H., Mattei, M. G., Sarfarazi, M., Tsipouras, P., Ramirez, F., and Hollister, D. W. (1991) *Nature* **352**, 330-334.

68. Maslen, C. L., Corson, G. M., Maddox, B. K., Glanville, R. W., and Sakai, L. Y. (1991) *Nature* **352**, 334-337.

69. Bode, W. and Schwager, P. (1975) *FEBS Lett.* **56**, 139-143.

70. Bode, W. and Schwager, P. (1975) *J. Mol. Biol.* **98**, 693-717.

71. Bajaj, S. P., Sabharwal, A. K., Gorka, J., and Birktoft, J. J. (1992) *Proc. Natl. Acad. Sci. USA* **89**, 152-156.

72. Bajaj, S. P., Rapaport, S. I., and Maki, S. L. (1985) *J. Biol. Chem.* **260**, 11574-11580.

73. Chattopadhyay, A., James, H. L., and Fair, D. S. (1992) *J. Biol. Chem.* **267**, 12323-12329.

74. Rezaie, A. R., Esmon, N. L., and Esmon, C. T. (1992) *J. Biol. Chem.* **267**, 11701-11704.

THROMBOMODULIN: ITS EXPRESSION AND RELEACE INTO THE CIRCULATION

Nobuo Aoki, Shin-ichi Ohdama, Kazunori Hirokawa
The First Department of Medicine, Tokyo Medical and Dental University, Yushima,
Bunkyo-Ku, Tokyo 113, Japan

Thrombomodulin(TM), is an endothelial cell surface glycoprotein that plays an important role in thromboresistance especially in microvasuculature. It forms a one to one complex with thrombin to inactivate its procoagulant property. This complex catalyzes activation of protein C and activated protein C inactivates coagulant factors Va and VIIIa in the presence of protein S. Thus, TM converts procoagulant thrombin to an anticoagulant and plays a central role in the protein C anticoagulant pathway. The physiological importance of the TM-protein C system in the prevention of thrombus formation is supported by various observations including thrombotic tendencies in patients with congenital deficiency of protein C and effective prevention of experimental thrombosis by intravenous administration of purified TM. Previous studies have shown that TM on endothelial cells is down-regulated by endotoxin, TNF or IL-1β. This loss of anticoagulant potential together with induction of tissue factor in blood coagulation by these agents is thought to be related to the hypercoagulative state of sepsis, chronic inflamation and cancer. Therefore, states of expression of TM on surfaces of endothelial cells are important in regulation of intravascular coagulation.

CELL SURFACE EXPRESSION OF TM

We have studied expression of TM on cultured human umbilical vein endothelial cells [1-5].
First, we confirmed the known effects of TNF and IL-1β on the cell surface TM activity. The cell surface TM activity was decreased dose-dependently by TNF, Lipopolysaccharide, LPS, extracted from E coli, synthetic lipid A possessing endotoxin activity, or IL-1β.
In contrast to these cytokines and endotoxins, cAMP analogs which increase intracellular cAMP, such as dibutyryl cAMP, 8-bromo cAMP and 8-(4-cyclophenylthio) cAMP, all increased the surface TM activity [1]. Further, an activator of adenylate cyclase, forskolin, which induces an increase of intracellular cAMP also increase surface TM activity on incubation. Since cGMP did not show any effect on TM activity [2], these results may suggest that protein kinase A is involved in the up-regulation of TM expression on cell surfaces. Among vasoactive amines, histamine also up-regulated cell surface TM via H_1-receptors [3]. Phorbol myristate acetate(PMA), exibited biphasic effects with reduced TM activity occurring between one to 6 hrs followed by a significant enhancement after 24 and 48 hrs incubation; that is down-regulation by short incubation and up-regulation by long incubation [2].
Effects of cycloheximide on cell surface TM activity were studied [1]. Incubation of cells with 1 to 10 μg/ml of cycloheximide did not change much of the cell surface TM activity. However, enhancement of TM activity by PMA or dibutyryl cAMP were both abolished by co-incubation with cycloheximide, indicating that the enhanced TM activity resulted from de novo synthesis of TM protein.
TNF induced remarkable reduction of TM mRNA. IL-1β also induced a similar time-depnedent decrease in TM mRNA. Dibutyryl cAMP increased TM mRNA between 2 to 4 hrs with maximal effect at 2h.
Phorbol ester, PMA, increased TM mRNA, reaching the maximum around 24 hrs incubation. There was no initial decrease of mRNA, which is contrary to the time course of surface TM activity in the cells stimulated by phorbol esters. Since down-regulation of TM by short incubation with phorbol ester, PMA, was not associated with decreased transcription, the initial decrease of surface TM activity may be caused by another mechanism such as internalization-degradation of the TM molecules.
To test such a possibility, we compared the time course of surface TM activity

14

and the total cellular TM antigen [2]. The results demonstrated that down-regulation of TM occurred initially on the cell surface followed by loss of antigen in the cells, and up-regulation occurred in reverse order. Analysis of TM antigen in culture media from these experiments did not show any significant change, indicating that faster decrease of surface TM as compared to the total cellular TM was not caused by release of TM into the media but may be caused by internalization of TM molecules into the cells and their subsequent degradation in the cells.

Down-regulation of surface TM by internalization and degradation of TM molecules in the cells was further indicated by the experiments with chloroquine. Chloroquine is known to inhibit lysozomal functions. Chloroquine did not cause any significant change of cell surface TM in the control cells and in the cells incubated with PMA, TNF or IL-1β for 4 hrs. However, the total cellular TM antigen was increased by the presence of chloroquine. This suggests that internalized TM molecules are subjected to lysozomal degradation.

Since dibutyryl cAMP and forskolin up-regulated surface TM activity, we have examined the effects of drugs which are known to increase intracellular cAMP on surface TM activity of endothelial cells. Pentoxifylline and theophylline at concentrations of 100 μg/ml increased surface TM approximately by 20% after 4 hrs incubation [4]. The increase of surface TM by pentoxifylline was associated with the increase of intracellular content of cAMP. Transcriptional levels for TM also increased by incubation of cells with pentoxifylline. The presence of pentoxifylline at concentrations of more than 10 μg/ml abrogated suppression of surface TM induced by 2 u/ml of TNF [4]. The result may indicate a plausable therapeutic application of pentoxifyline in prevention of thrombosis particularly associated with infection, since up-regulation of surface TM was observed with more than 1 μg/ml of pentoxifyline, and 1 to 3 μg/ml plasma are therapeutic concentrations obtained by usual doses of pentoxifyline.

Retinoic acid, one of the metabolites of vitamin A, is a regulatory compound involved in cell proliferation and differentiation. Trans-form of retinoic acid was found to increase the cell surface TM; one μM of retinoic acid increased surface TM approximately to 150% [5]. The retinoic acid concentrations effective in up-regulation of surface TM were well in the range of therapeutic plasma concentrations achieved in the treatment of acute promyelocytic leukemia with retinoic acid, suggesting clinical application of retinoic acid in prevention and treatment of disseminated intravascular coagulation associated with various diseases.

PLASMA TM

Although TM is mainly present on endothelial cell surfaces, TM is also found in circulating blood plasma. We have examined TM present in plasma using three kinds of monoclonal antibodies to human TM [6]. The results showed that plasma TM consists of 4 major forms and their molcular weights are smaller than that of intact TM purified from tissues. Normal plasma contains approximately 10 ng/ml of TM on average measured by enzyme-linked immunosorbent assay. In various disease states such as intravascular coagulation, adult respiratory distress syndrome, pulmonary thromboembolism, chronic renal failure and acute hepatic failure, plasma TM levels were significantly elevated. The increase of plasma TM found in these patients was mainly due to an increase of the smaller fragments of degraded forms. This suggests that the release of TM from endothelial cells was accelerated in various disease states by proteolytic activity generated on the surface of the endothelium. Elevated levels of plasma TM in chronic renal failure and acute hepatic failure may suggest that plasma TM may be removed from the circulation mostly by the kidneys and liver.

Recently, we found that plasma TM levels are elevated in systemic lupus erythematosus, rheumatoid arthritis, and Behcet disease, when these diseases are active. The highest value obtained in active SLE was nearly 20 times of the normal control. When these disease states are inactive, the plasma TM levels are not significantly different from the normal control.

In the other collagen diseases, progressive systemic slerosis, polymyositis-dermatomyositis, and Wegeners's granulomatosis, showed significantly elevated values. In Wegener's granulomatosis, the plasma TM levels correlated with the extent of pulmonary lesion. These results all together may indicate that plasma TM can be used as a marker for endothelial cell injuries.

CONCLUSION

In conclusion, endothelial cell surface TM is regulated by various agents. It is down-regulated by TNF, IL-1β, endotoxins and phorbol esters on short incubation, and is up-regulated by cAMP, histamine, retinoic acid and phorbol esters on long incubation. These modulations of TM expression on endothelial cell surfaces are achieved by independent mechanisms causing a change of transcriptional rate and internalization-degradation of the molecules. The mechanisms may involve protein kinase A and protein kinase C. Degraded forms of TM are found in circulating blood plasma, and these molecules may have been released from endothelial cell surfaces by proteolytic activity generated on endothelium in various diseases. Plasma TM may be considered to be a valuable marker for endothelial cell injuries.

REFERENCES

1. Hirokawa K, Aoki N (1990) Up-regulation of thrombomodulin in human umbilical vein endothelial cells in vitro. J Biochem 108:839-845

2. Hirokawa K, Aoki N (1991) Regulatory mechanisms for thrombomodulin expression in human umbilical vein endothelial cells in vitro. J Cell Physiol 147:157-165

3. Hirokawa K, Aoki N (1991) Up-regulation of thrombomodulin by activation of histamine H_1-receptors in human umbilical-vein endothelial cells in vitro. Biochem J 276:739-743

4. Ohdama S, Takano S, Ohashi K, Miyake S, Aoki N (1991) Pentoxifylline prevents tumor necrosis factor-induced suppression of endothelial cell surface thrombomodulin. Thromb Res 62:745-755

5. Miyake S, Ohdama S, Tazawa R, Aoki N (1992) Retinoic acid prevents cytokine-induced suppression of thrombomodulin expression on surface of human vascular endtothelial cells in vitro. Thromb Res in press

6. Takano S, Kimura S, Ohdama S, Aoki N (1990) Plasma thrombomodulin in health and diseases. Blood 76:2024-2029

RECOGNITION SITES FOR THROMBOMODULIN, PROCOAGULANT AND ANTICOAGULANT PROTEINS AROUND THE ACTIVE CENTER OF THROMBIN

KOJI SUZUKI AND JUNJI NISHIOKA

Department of Molecular Biology on Genetic Disease, Mie University School of Medicine, Tsu-city, Mie 514, Japan

INTRODUCTION

Thrombin (α-thrombin) is a multifunctional serine protease that functions in hemostasis by acting on many plasma procoagulant proteins, fibrinogen, Factor V and platelets. When thrombin binds to thrombomodulin (TM), a receptor on the vascular endothelial cells [1,2], thrombin acts on the plasma anticoagulant protein C [1,3], thereby completely diminishing its ability to activate the procoagulant proteins [4-6]. On the mechanism of this conversion of the thrombin substrate specificity, on one hand, TM is suggested to induce a conformational change in the active center of thrombin [7,8]. On the other hand, we found that TM bound to a region involving the sequence residues Thr-147 to Ser-158 of the B-chain of thrombin [9] and a peptide TWTANVGKGQPS corresponding to these residues inhibited the thrombin-induced fibrinogen clotting, Factor V activation and platelet activation as well as thrombin binding to TM [10]. Recent crystallographic studies revealed that thrombin is composed of several module structures around its active center [11,12], and one of the modules was realized to correspond to the region involving the residues Thr-147 to Ser-158. In this study, to elucidate the functional role of the modules of thrombin, particularly related to the mechanism of the TM-induced conversion of thrombin substrate specificity, we synthesized several peptides corresponding to the module structures, and studied their effects on the interaction of thrombin with TM, and procoagulant and anticoagulant proteins.

MATERIALS AND METHODS

Proteins and Reagents - All chemicals were of the highest commercial grade avail-

---

Key words: Thrombin, Thrombomodulin, Protein C, Fibrinogen, Factor V

able. Protein C, thrombin, Factor V, prothrombin, Factor X, fibrinogen, antithrombin III, recombinant TM and hirudin were all purified from human plasma, cultured
medium of the mammalian cells or obtained commercially available as described
[9,10]. The chromogenic substrates for activated protein C, S-2366, and for thrombin, S-2238, were obtained from Kabi, Sweden.

Preparation of Peptides - Peptides, FRKSPQELL, LLYPPWDKNF, RIGKHSRTRYER, LEKIYIHP,
RYNWREN, TWTANVGKGQPS, DSTRIRI, EGDSGGP, and SWGEGCDRDGK, respectively corresponding
to sequence residues Phe-19 to Leu-27, Leu-45 to Phe-53, Arg-62 to Arg-73, Leu-81 to
Pro-88, Arg-89 to Asn-95, Thr-147 to Ser-158, Asp-175 to Ile-181, Glu-202 to Pro-
208, and Ser-226 to Lys-236 of B-chain of thrombin, which are the module structures
located on the surface and around the active center of thrombin [11] were prepared
using an Applied Biosystems Model 431A peptide synthesizer and then purified by
reversed phase HPLC [10].   Peptides, NERWNYR and SPQGKGVNATWT, respectively corresponding to the inverted sequence residues of Leu-89 to Asn-95 and Thr-147 to Ser-
158, were prepared by the same method.

Assay of Peptide Effects on Thrombin Functions - Binding of thrombin to TM fixed in
microwell plates (CO-BIND, Micro Membranes) and apparent inhibition constants (K_i)
of peptides in the thrombin TM interaction were determined [9,10].

Binding of TM to the peptides was determined as follows: Each peptide was
immobilized to microwell plates using a Peptide coating Kit (Takara-Biochemicals).
To the peptide-coated microwells, TM was added and incubated.   After washing the
wells, protein C and thrombin were added to the wells, and the activated protein C
was determined using S-2366.

Effects of the peptides on thrombin-catalyzed protein C activation, thrombin-
induced fibrinogen clotting and Factor V activation, thrombin inhibition by antithrombin III and by hirudin were determined basically as described previously [10].

RESULTS

Effects of Peptides on Thrombin Binding to Thrombomodulin - Of the peptides tested,
100 μM TWTANVGKGQPS, RYNWREN and LLYPPWDKNF inhibited thrombin binding to TM, and
the two former peptides inhibited the binding in proportion to the peptide concentration (**Fig.1**). The inhibitory effect of LLYPPWDKNF appeared to diminish at higher

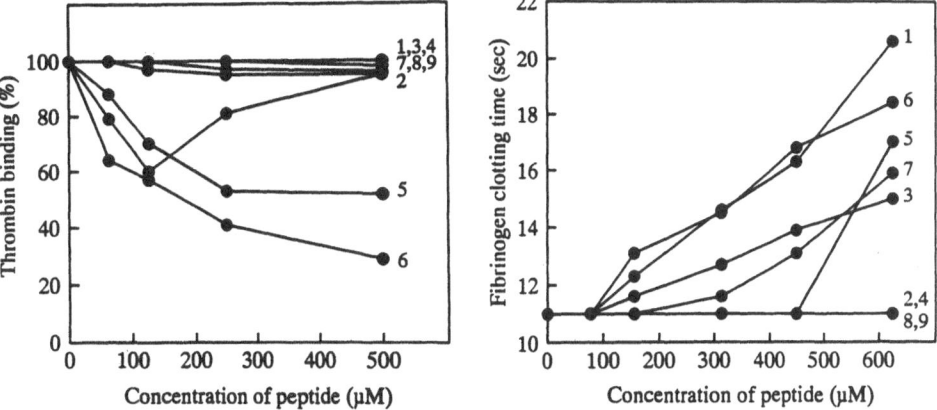

Fig. 1 Effects of thrombin-based peptides on thrombin binding to TM. A mixture of thrombin and various concentrations of peptide (indicated as final concentrations) was added to microwells containing fixed TM. After washing the wells, the thrombin bound to the wells was determined using S-2238. The activity of the bound thrombin without peptide was assigned as 100%. 1, FRKSPQELL; 2, LLYPPWDKNF; 3, RIGKHSRTRYER; 4, LEKIYIHP; 5, RYNWREN; 6, TWTANVGKGQPS; 7, DSTRIRI; 8, EGDSGGP; 9, SWGEGCDRDGK

Fig. 2 Effects of thrombin-based peptides on thrombin-induced fibrinogen clotting. To a mixture of thrombin and various concentrations of peptide (indicated as final concentrations), fibrinogen was added and the clotting time was determined. Peptide Nos. are noted in the legend to Fig. 1.

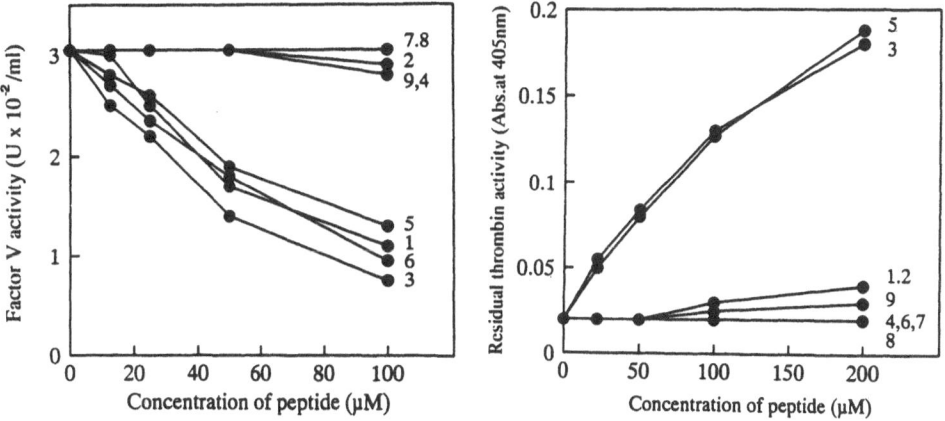

Fig. 3. Effects of thrombin-based peptides on thrombin-induced Factor V activation. A mixture of Factor V and various concentrations of peptide (indicated as final concentrations) was incubated with thrombin. To this mixture, were added prothrombin and rabbit brain cephalin, then Factor Xa. After a 5-min incubation, generated thrombin was determined using S-2238. Peptide Nos. are noted in the legend to Fig. 1.

Fig. 4. Effects of thrombin-based peptides on thrombin inhibition by antithrombin III. A mixture of antithrombin III and various concentrations of peptide (indicated as final concentrations) was incubated with thrombin (0.02 U) for 15 min, and the residual thrombin activity was determined using S-2238. Peptide Nos. are noted in the legend to Fig. 1.

concentrations. The apparent inhibition constants ($\underline{Ki}$) of TWTANVGKGQPS and RYNWREN for thrombin binding to TM were 97 and 80 μM, respectively. Both of the peptides with the inverted sequence of TWTANVGKGQPS and RYNWREN did not inhibit thrombin binding to TM (data not shown). The inhibitory effects of TWTANVGKGQPS and RYNWREN upon thrombin binding to TM were additive (data not shown). TM also bound directly to the two peptides depending on the amount of the peptide fixed in microwells (data not shown).

Effect of Peptides on Protein C Activation by Thrombin - Only a peptide, EGDSGGP, of the tested peptides inhibited the protein C activation in the absence of TM and Ca^{2+} ions (data not shown).

Effect of peptides on Thrombin-induced Fibrinogen Clotting - Peptides, FRKSPQELL, TWTANVGKGQPS, RIGKHSRTRYER and DSTRIRI effectively prolonged the clotting time in proportion to the peptide concentration, and RYNWREN also prolonged the clotting time at higher concentrations (**Fig.2**). The concentration of half-maximal inhibition caused by FRKSPQELL and TWTANVGKGQPS for thrombin-induced fibrinogen clotting were 360 and 385 μM, respectively. Inhibition constants for RIGKHSRTRYER, RYNWREN and DSTRIRI were unobtainable, since inhibition by these peptides was unsaturable.

Effects of Peptide on Thrombin-induced Factor V Activation - FRKSPQELL, RIGKHSRTRYER, RYNWREN and TWTANVGKGQPS markedly inhibited thrombin-induced Factor V activation in proportion to the peptide concentration (**Fig.3**). The apparent inhibition constants for thrombin-induced Factor V activation of FRKSPQELL, RIGKHSRTRYER, RYNWREN and TWTANVGKGQPS were 71, 143, 42 and 83 μM, respectively.

Effects of Peptides on Inhibition of Thrombin by Antithrombin III or Hirudin - Peptides, RIGKHSRTRYER and RYNWREN specifically blocked the inhibition of thrombin by antithrombin III in the absence of heparin (**Fig. 4**). The apparent inhibition constants of the respective peptides for the inhibition were 111 and 100 μM, respectively. Peptides, RIGKHSRTRYER, FRKSPQELL and TWTANVGKGQPS, in that order, specifically blocked the inhibition of the amidolytic activity of thrombin by hirudin in proportion to the peptide concentration (data not sown). The inhibition constants of the three peptides in blocking the thrombin inhibition by hirudin were not obtained, since the inhibition was unsaturable.

DISCUSSION

In the present study, we found that, in addition to the peptide TWTANVGKGQPS, another peptide RYNWREN inhibited thrombin binding to TM. The inhibitory effects of the two peptides were additive, and TM directly bound to the two peptides. Moreover, LLYPPWDKNF appeared to inhibit the thrombin TM interaction with an optimal concentration of 100 μM, although the manner of inhibition was unclear. These results suggest that there are at least three interactive sites for TM to thrombin. Recently, Ye et al.[13] suggested the presence of at least two interaction sites for TM in thrombin. The first site is located at a region immediately adjacent to the active Ser residue of thrombin and the second site is located at a region considerably further than 15 A from the active Ser residue. Although at present we do not define which region suggested by Ye et al. corresponds to the two interaction sites in thrombin that we found in this study.

Furthermore, this study suggested that the module structures around the active center of thrombin play a role in the interaction with several procoagulant and anticoagulant substrates. Protein C interacts with the region consisting of the residues Glu-202 to Pro-208, which contains a Ser residue in the active center pocket. Fibrinogen interacts relatively strongly with regions Phe-19 to Leu-27 and Thr-147 to Ser-158, and moderately with region Arg-62 to Arg-73, termed an anion-binding exosite, and moreover, weakly with the regions Asp-175 to Ile-181 and Arg-89 to Asn-95. Factor V strongly interacts with the four regions Phe-19 to Leu-27, Arg-62 to Arg-73, Arg-89 to Asn-95 and Thr-147 to Ser-158. Antithrombin III definitely interacts with two regions consisting of residues Arg-62 to Arg-73 and Arg-89 to Asn-95. Hirudin strongly interacts in the following order with regions Arg-62 to Arg-73, Phe-19 to Leu-27 and Thr-147 to Ser-158. These data also indicate that a protein substrate interacts with at least two or more sites on the surface of thrombin, and that a region on the surface of thrombin molecule serves as the interaction site for several substrates.

These findings suggest that TM interacts with at least three sites around the active center of thrombin, and these sites are shared in part with the recognition sites for procoagulant and/or anticoagulant substrates except for protein C. This may lead a reason that TM blocks the activation of procoagulant substrates by thrombin and selectively activates protein C, in addition to another reason that TM induces the conformational change of the active center of thrombin as suggested by Ye et al..

Acknowledgement - We thank Dr. Bode W. in Max-Plank Institute providing us the data on the crystal structure of α-thrombin, and also Dr. Toma K. helping us to analyze those data.

REFERENCES

1. Esmon NL, Owen WG, Esmon CT (1982) J Biol Chem 257: 859-864

2. Suzuki K, Kusumoto H, Deyashiki Y, Nishioka J, Maruyama I, Zushi M, Kawahara S, Honda G, Yamamoto S, Horiguchi S (1987) EMBO J 6: 1891-1897

3. Esmon CT (1989) J Biol Chem 264: 4743-4746

4. Esmon CT, Esmon NL, Harris KW (1983) J Biol Chem 258: 7944-7947

5. Esmon NL, Carroll RC, Esmon CT (1983) J Biol Chem 258: 12238-12242

6. Suzuki K, Stenflo J, Dahlback B, Teodorsson B (1983) J Biol Chem 258: 1914-1920

7. Esmon CT, Esmon NL, Kurosawa S, Johnson AE (1986) Ann N Y Acad Sci 485: 215-220

8. Musci G, Berliner LJ, Esmon CT (1988) Biochemistry 27: 769-773

9. Suzuki K, Nishioka J, Hayashi T (1990) J Biol Chem 265: 13263-13267

10. Suzuki K, Nishioka J (1991) J Biol Chem 266: 18498-18501

11. Bode W, Mayr I, Baumann U, Huber R, Stone SR, Hofsteenge J (1989) EMBO J 8: 3467-3475

12. Grutter MG, Priestle JP, Rahuel J, Grossenbacher H, Bode W, Hofsteenge J, Stone R (1990) EMBO J 9: 2361-2365

13. Ye J, Esmon NL, Esmon CT, Johnson AE (1991) J Biol Chem 266: 23016-23021

HEPARIN-BINDING SITE(S) OF ANTITHROMBIN III, HISTIDINE-RICH GLYCOPROTEIN AND ACTIVATED PROTEIN C

T. Koide

Department of Life Science, Faculty of Science, Himeji Institute of Technology, Kamigori, Hyogo 678-12, Japan.

INTRODUCTION

Many plasma proteins associated with the regulation and modulation of blood coagulation and fibrinolysis are known to function through the interaction with heparin. These include antithrombin III (ATIII), heparin cofactor II, protein C inhibitor, plasminogen activator inhibitor 1, tissue factor pathway inhibitor, histidine-rich glycoprotein (HRG), vitronectin, thrombospondin and platelet factor 4. In addition, recently, we found that activated protein C (APC), an important anticoagulant protease, has a high affinity for heparin. In this brief communication, I will summarize our investigations on the heparin-binding site(s) of ATIII, HRG and APC, and discuss them together with those of other heparin-binding plasma proteins whether or not there is any common feature of the heparin-binding sequences among these proteins.

1. HEPARIN-BINDING SITE(S) OF ANTITHROMBIN III (ATIII)

ATIII is a single chain glycoprotein of Mr 59,000 that plays the most important role in the regulation of blood coagulation, capable of inhibiting thrombin, factor Xa and factor IXa. The characteristic feature of ATIII is that the protease inhibitory activity of ATIII is enhanced a few thousand-fold in the presence of heparin. The amino acid sequence of ATIII composed of 432 residues has been determined both by peptide [1] and by DNA [2-4] sequencings. The heparin-binding site(s) of ATIII have been studied from various aspects, which include the structural analysis of hereditary abnormal molecule that is defective in the heparin-binding, chemical and enzymatic degradations, followed by the isolation of the heparin-binding fragment(s), characterization of recombinant variants or fragments, and synthesis and elucidation of the heparin-binding peptide.

Physiological importance of the heparin-binding ability of ATIII is well demonstrated by many cases of thrombosis caused by a hereditary abnormal ATIII whose heparin-binding ability is lost. A typical case of such abnormal ATIII is ATIII-Toyama, whose molecular abnormality we have identified as an Arg47 to Cys substitution by a detailed structural analysis of abnormal protein in 1984 [5]. In the following years, many natural mutants of Arg47 have been characterized [6-9], all of which are defective in the heparin-binding, giving the increasing evidence that Arg47 is one of the integral residues in ATIII for the interaction with heparin. Besides Arg47, several new variants of other residues with defective heparin-binding have been characterized (see for database [10]). It should be noted that the mutation sites of all variants of heparin-binding defects are located in the N-terminal region of the polypeptide. To support this, a recombinant ATIII mutant, devoid of amino acid residues 41-49, was shown to have decreased heparin-binding and two truncated forms of ATIII, one consisting of residues 219-432 and the other consisting of residues 251-432, were shown not to bind to heparin [11]. On the other hand, chemical modification studies have shown that Lys107 [12], Lys114 [13], Lys125 [12, 13, 14], Arg129 [15] Lys136 [12] and Arg145 [15] are involved in the interaction of ATIII with heparin. The heparin-binding peptide corresponding to residues 114-156 was isolated [16] and a synthetic peptide, consisting of residues 123-139 was shown to bind heparin and inhibit the binding of ATIII and heparin [17]. Furthermore, polyclonal antibody raised against a synthetic peptide corresponding to residues 124-145 in human ATIII was shown to specifically block the binding of heparin to ATIII [18].

Taken together, it would be concluded that the heparin-binding site(s) of ATIII comprise two regions, helices A and D, of the polypeptide chain; namely, Arg47 [5, 8, 9] in helix A and basic amino acid residues in helix D including Lys125 [12, 13, 14], Arg129 [15, 19], Arg132, Arg133 and Lys136 [12], together with Lys107 [12], Lys114 [13] and Arg145 [15]. The amino acid residues involved in the heparin-binding of ATIII are collectively illustrated in **Fig.1**. All of these basic residues are conserved among human [1-4], bovine [20], rabbit [21] and porcine (Koide, T., unpublished result) ATIII (**Fig. 2**).

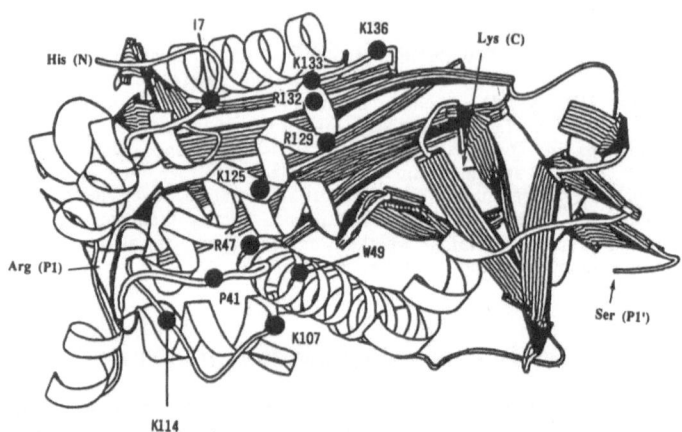

Fig. 1. Ribbon schematic representation of ATIII (Taken from L. Mourey *et al.* [22] with permission and some modifications were added). The amino acid residues involved in the heparin-binding are shown in solid circles with one letter symbols and residue numbers from the N-terminus of human ATIII. His (N) and Lys (C) indicate the N-terminal and the C-terminal residues, respectively. Arg (P1) and Ser (P1') indicate the reactive site residues whose peptide bond has been cleaved.

```
          101      ▼          ▼   120  ▼  ▼      ▼  140   ▼   150
Human     QLMEVFKFDT ISEKTSDQIH FFFAKLNCRL YRKANKSSKL VSANRLFGDK
Bovine    ---------- ---------- ---------- --------E- ----------
Porcine   -------- --------V- ---------- --------E- ----------
Rabbit    ---------- --------V- ---------- ---------- ----------
Mouse     ---------- ---------- ---------- --------D- ----------
```

Fig. 2. Comparison of the amino acid sequences of five ATIIIs in the heparin-binding region. Those residues identical to human species are shown by bars. All the amino acid residues involved in the heparin-binding (shown by arrowheads) are conserved among five ATIIIs. Arg47 (not shown in the figure) is also conserved among these ATIIIs. Residue numbering is that of human ATIII.

2.   HEPARIN-BINDING SITE(S) OF HISTIDINE-RICH GLYCOPROTEIN (HRG)

Heparin-dependent thrombin inhibition of ATIII can be neutralized by histidine-rich glycoprotein (HRG), another plasma protein with a high affinity for heparin. The glycoprotein, thereby, can be isolated together with ATIII by heparin-agarose affinity chromatography [23].   HRG is a single chain glycoprotein of Mr 67,000, exceptionally rich in histidine and proline residues [24].   Besides the interaction with heparin, a number of biological properties have been reported for HRG, which includes interactions with plasmin(ogen), fibrin(ogen), thrombospondin, activated platelets, T-lymphocytes and monocytes (see for review [25]).   Although the physiological role of HRG is not definitely established yet, a high risk of thrombosis in families with elevated levels of HRG [26]

strongly suggests that the heparin-binding property of HRG is physiologically significant.
The polypeptide is composed of several consecutive structural domains, including the N-terminal two cystatin (cysteine protease inhibitor)-like domains, followed by a histidine-rich domain which is preceded and followed by two proline-rich domains [24].

We have studied the heparin-binding site of HRG by a limited proteolysis with chymotrypsin, followed by the isolation of the potent heparin-binding fragment(s). The SDS-polyacrylamide gel electrophoresis pattern (reduced) of the chymotrypsin digest showed that the 35/38 kDa doublet bands which are produced as early as after the 5-min digestion were stable even after the 60-min digestion, and when applied to a heparin-agarose column, these fragments were recovered from the column only after the elution with a buffer containing as high as 2M NaCl, which is equivalent to the salt concentration to elute native HRG. The amino acid composition and N-terminal sequence analyses of the isolated heparin-binding fragment(s) indicated that the heparin-binding site of HRG is located within the N-terminal two cystatin-like domains. Since the cystatin-like domain is very resistant to a further digestion by chymotrypsin, we could not determine a more specific heparin-binding site within the region. To support this result, however, this region contains the segments whose sequences are homologous to those of the heparin-binding sites of ATIII, heparin cofactor II (HCII) (see Fig. 6) and von Willebrand factor (vWF) [27] (**Fig. 3**). It should be noted that most of the basic residues important for the heparin-binding of AT III and HC II are also conserved in HRG [28]. Thus, we tentatively propose that the heparin-binding site of HRG is formed by a region consisting of residues 72-146 which is very similar, not quite identical to those of ATIII and HCII, and partly homologous to that of vWF.

A T III	Thr (44)	Asn	Arg	Arg (47)	Val	Trp	Glu	Leu	Ser	Lys	Ala	Asn	Ser (56)
H R G	Asp (76)	Ser	Arg	Arg	Pro	Ser	Glu	Ile	Val	Ile	Gly	Gln	Cys (87)
v W F	Asp (570)	Arg	Lys	Arg	Pro	Ser	Glu	Leu	Arg	Arg	Ile	Ala	Ser (582)

Fig. 3. Comparison of the partial amino acid sequence of HRG with those of the heparin-binding regions of ATIII and vWF. Conserved amino acid residues are shown in blocks.

3. HEPARIN-BINDING SITE OF ACTIVATED PROTEIN C (APC)

Protein C (PC) is a zymogen form of a vitamin-K dependent serine protease present in plasma. It is activated by a thrombin-thrombomodulin complex on the endothelial cell surface, and activated protein C (APC) functions as a regulator of blood coagulation by inactivating factors Va and VIIIa, and also as a stimulator of fibrinolysis by inactivating plasminogen activator inhibitor 1 (see for review [29]).
Protein C is composed of two polypeptide-chains. The N-terminal light chain consists of Gla domain and two epidermal growth factor (EGF)-like domains, and the C-terminal heavy chain consists of activation peptide and catalytic domain.
In course of the study of neutralization by HRG of the heparin-dependent activity of protein C inhibitor to inhibit APC, we found that APC shows a high affinity for heparin, which is enhanced in the presence of Ca^{2+}, although Ca^{2+} is not essential for the interaction between heparin and APC (**Fig.4**).
In order to examine the contribution of Gla domain to the heparin-binding property of protein C and APC, Gla domainless (GD) protein C was prepared by limited proteolysis with chymotrypsin, then GD-APC was prepared by the activation of GD-protein C with a thrombin-thrombomodulin complex. As shown in Fig.4, both GD-protein C and GD-APC retained the same affinity as protein C and APC, respectively, for heparin. Furthermore, GD-APC showed the same Ca^{2+}-dependent augment as APC in its heparin binding. Thus, Gla domain of APC was shown not to be involved in the interaction with heparin.

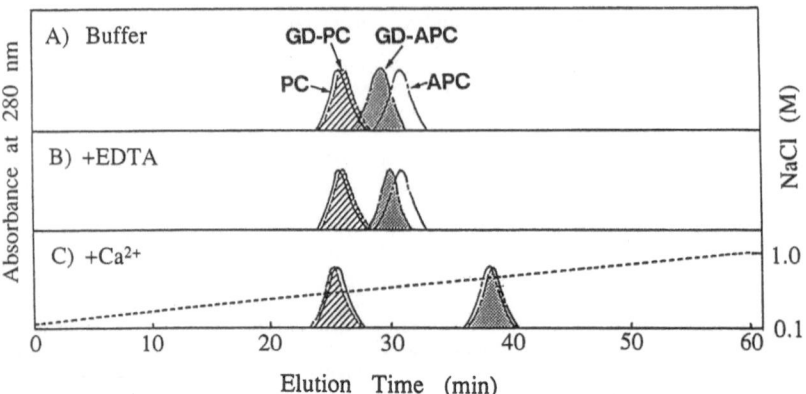

Fig. 4 Heparin-binding abilities of protein C, APC, and their Gla domainless derivatives. Heparin-Sepharose chromatography was performed at 25 °C using a column (0.5 x 10 cm) mounted on an FPLC system (Pharmacia). The column was equilibrated with, A) 50 mM Tris-0.1 M NaCl, pH7.4, B) 50 mM Tris-0.1 M NaCl, pH7.4, containing 20 μM EDTA, or C) 50 mM Tris-0.1 M NaCl, pH7.4, containing 1 mM CaCl$_2$. Each protein was applied separately and eluted with a linear gradient of NaCl concentration (0.1-1.0 M in 60 min) at a flow rate of 0.2 ml/min. The elution time indicates the time after a gradient elution was started. The height and shape of each protein peak is arbitrary.

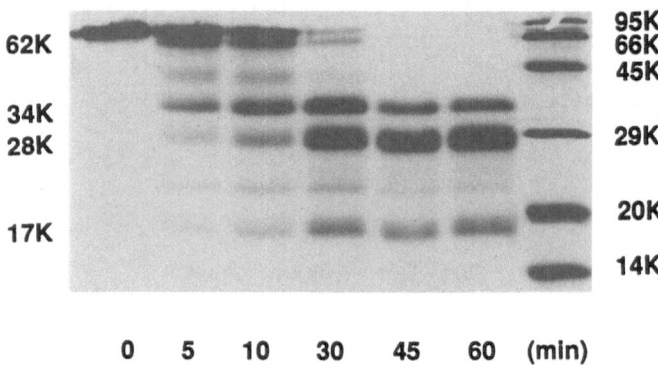

0   5   10   30   45   60   (min)

Fig. 5.   Limited proteolysis of protein C with Sepharose-bound trypsin. Protein C was digested at 4 °C with Sepharose-bound trypsin. Aliquots of samples were withdrawn at different intervals and subjected to SDS-10% polyacrylamide gel electrophoresis without reducing agents. The lane on the right hand side shows the standard molecular markers.

The heparin-binding site of APC was further studied by a limited proteolysis with Sepharose-bound trypsin, followed by the isolation and characterization of the heparin-binding fragment. A digestion of native protein C with Sepharose-bound trypsin time-dependently produced degradation products of Mr 34kDa, 28kDa and 17kDa (**Fig.5**). A 60-min digest was incubated overnight at 4 °C with heparin-Sepharose, equilibrated with 50 mM Tris-HCl, pH 7.4 and 50 mM NaCl, in the presence or absence of 1 mM Ca^{2+}. Heparin-Sepharose was then packed into the FPLC column (HR 5/10). After removing unbound materials by washing the column with the equilibration buffer, the 34 kDa fragment was eluted from the column at salt concentrations of 0.53 M and 0.68 M in the absence and presence of 1 mM Ca^{2+}, respectively, which are exactly the same as those of APC and GD-APC (Fig. 4).

From the N-terminal amino acid sequence and the amino acid composition analyses of the isolated fragments, the 34K heparin-binding fragment was identified to consist of two EGF domains (His44 to Lys146) and the N-terminal portion of the heavy-chain of APC (Leu1 to Arg145 or Lys153). Another large fragment, the 28K heparin-*non*binding fragment was identified to consist of two EGF domains (His44 to Lys146) and the N-terminal truncated heavy-chain (Trp62 or Trp65 to Arg145 or Lys153). These results indicate that the 28K fragment was produced from the 34K fragment by further tryptic hydrolysis of an Arg61-Trp (or Lys64-Trp) bond. From these results, it is highly likely that the heparin-binding site of APC is involved in the N-terminal region (Leu1 to Arg61) of the heavy-chain. This region is extremely rich in basic residues when compared with those of other vitamin K-dependent coagulation factors. Furthermore, this region contains Lys5-Met-Thr-Arg-Arg and Lys48-Lys-Leu-Leu-Val-Arg sequences that are common features of the heparin-binding sequences of many heparin-binding plasma proteins as shown in **Fig.6**.

A computer simulation model of the protease domain of human APC reveals that the side-chains of basic amino acid residues in the putative heparin-binding region are located on the surface of the molecule (unpublished result).

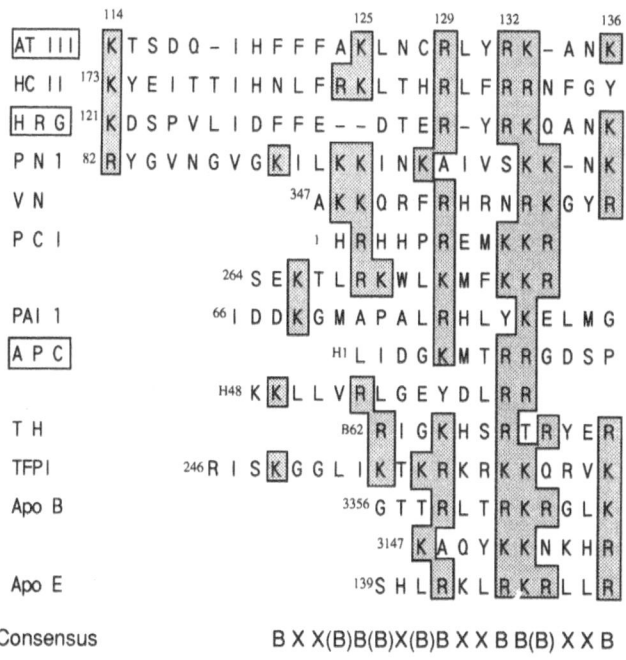

Fig. 6.   Proposed heparin-binding sites of activated protein C, together with those of heparin-binding proteins in human plasma. Common basic amino acid residues are shown in shaded blocks. ATIII, antithrombin III;   HCII, heparin cofactor II;   HRG, histidine-rich glycoprotein;   PN1, protease nexin 1;   VN, vitronectin;   PCI, protein C inhibitor;   PAI 1, plasminogen activator inhibitor 1;   APC, activated protein C;   TH, thrombin;   TFPI, tissue factor pathway inhibitor;   Apo B, apolipoprotein B-100;   Apo E, apolipoprotein E. Letters B, X, and (B) of consensus sequence indicate basic residue, any residue, and less frequently occurring basic residue, respectively.

ACKNOWLEDGEMENTS

The author thanks Dr Yoshiaki Kazama for his collaboration in the study of heparin-binding site of APC. Thanks are also to Dr. Walter Kisiel for his kind supply of protein C. This work was supported in part by a Grant-in-Aid for Scientific Research (01480298) and a Grant-in-Aid for Scientific Research on Priority Areas (63616512) from the Ministry of Education, Science, and Culture of Japan.

REFERENCES

1. Petersen TE, Dudek-Wojciechowska G, Sottrup-Jensen L, Magnusson S (1979) In: Collen D, Wiman B, Verstraete M (eds) The Physiological Inhibitors of Blood Coagulation and Fibrinolysis. Elsevier. Amsterdam. pp43-54.
2. Bock SC, Wion KL, Vehar GA, Lawn RM (1982) Nucleic Acids Res. 10: 8113-8125
3. Chandra T, Stackhouse R, Kidd VJ, Woo SLC (1983) Proc. Natl. Acad. Sci., USA 80: 1845-1848
4. Prochownik EW, Markham AF, Orkin SH (1983) J. Biol. Chem., 258: 8389-8394
5. Koide T, Odani S, Takahashi K, Ono Y, Sakuragawa N (1984)   Proc. Natl. Acad. Sci., USA 81: 289-293
6. Duchange F, Chassé J-F, Cohen GN, Zakin MM (1987) Thromb. Res., 45: 115-121
7. Brunel F, Duchange N, Fischer A-M, Cohen GN, Zakin MM (1987) Am. J. Hematol., 25: 223-224
8. Owen MC, Borg JY, Soria C, Soria J, Caen J, Carrell RW (1987) Blood 69: 1275-1279
9. Borg JY, Owen MC, Soria C, Soria J, Caen J, Carrell RW (1988) J. Clin. Invest., 81: 1292-1296
10. Lane DA, Ireland H, Olds RJ, Thein SL, Perry DJ, Aiach M (1991) Thromb. Haemostas., 66: 657-661
11. Austin RC, Sheffield WP, Rachubinski RA, Blajchman MA (1992) Biochem. J., 282: 345-351
12. Chang JY (1989) J. Biol. Chem., 264: 3111-3115
13. Liu CS, Chang JY (1987) J. Biol. Chem., 262: 17356-17361
14. Peterson CB, Noyes CM, Pecon JM, Church FC, Blackburn MN (1987) J. Biol. Chem., 262: 8061-8065
15. Sun XJ, Chang JY (1990) Biochemistry, 29: 8957-8962
16. Smith JW, Knauer DJ (1987) J. Biol. Chem., 262: 11964-11972
17. Coffman Lellouch A, Lansbury PT Jr. (1992) Biochemistry 31: 2279-2285
18. Smith JW, Dey N, Knauer DJ (1990) Biochemistry, 29: 8950-8957
19. Gandrille S, Aiach M, Lane DA, Vidaud D, Molho-Sabatier P, Caso R, de Moerloose P, Fiessinger JN, Clauser E (1990) J. Biol. Chem., 265: 18997-19001
20. Mejdoub H, Le Ret M, Boulanger Y, Maman M, Choay J, Reinbolt J (1991) J. Protein Chem., 10: 205-212
21. Sheffield WP, Brothers AB, Wells MJ, Hatton MWC, Clarke BJ, Blajchman MA (1992) Blood 79: 2330-2339
22. Mourey L, Samama JP, Delarue M, Choay J, Lormeau JC, Petitou M, Moras D (1990) Biochimie 72: 599-608
23. Koide T, Odani S, Ono T (1985) J. Biochem (Tokyo) 98: 1191-1200
24. Koide T, Foster D, Yoshitake S, Davie EW (1986) Biochemistry, 25: 2220-2225
25. Koide T (1988) In: Gaffney PJ, Castellino FJ, Plow EF, Takada A (eds) Fibrinolysis. Current Prospects. John Libbey. London. pp55-63.
26. Engesser L, Kluft C, Briet E, Brommer EJP (1987) Brit. J. Haematol. 67: 355-358
27. Sobel M, Soler DF, Kermode JC, Harris RB (1992) J. Biol. Chem. 267: 8857-8862
28. Koide T, Foster D, Odani S (1986) FEBS Lett. 194: 242-244
29. Esmon CT (1989) J. Biol. Chem. 264: 4743-4746

THE CLEAVAGE OF A SERINE PROTEASE INHIBITOR AT THE REACTIVE CENTER BY ITS TARGET PROTEASE: ANALYSIS OF THE SUBSTRATE-LIKE FORM OF A SERPIN.

Tetsumei Urano, Kiyohito Serizawa, Kenji Sakakibara, Leif Strandberg*,
Tor Ny*, Yumiko Takada and Akikazu Takada
Department of Physiology, Hamamatsu University School of Medicine, Handa-cho, Hamamatsu, 431-31, Japan and Department of Applied Cell and Molecular Biology*, Umeå University, S-901 87 Umeå, Sweden

INTRODUCTION

Many enzymes involved in coagulation and fibrinolysis have a serine residue at their active site and they are therefore defined as serine proteases. In plasma the activity of such proteases are controlled by specific inhibitors belonging to the serine protease inhibitor (SERPIN) family that forms stoichiometric tight complexes with the target proteases. The inhibitors of the SERPIN family are thought to have a common tertiary structure[1] with a reactive center located on an exposed loop denoted "the strained loop", situated near the carboxyl terminus of the inhibitor molecule[2-4]. These inhibitors interact with their target proteases by providing a so called "bait" residue (P1 residue), that mimics the normal substrate of the target proteases[2,3,5]. The complex is supposed to exist either as Michaelis type, tetrahedral type[6,7] or acylintermediate[8,9], although which stage is the stable state is not clear. Recently, we discovered that the SERPIN plasminogen activator inhibitor 1 (PAI-1) can be cleaved by plasminogen activators at its reactive site and that treatment with low concentrations of sodium dodecyl sulphate (SDS) converts active PAI-1 to a form that is cleaved like a substrate[10]. Since the conformation of the cleavable PAI-1 is completely different from its native form we defined it as the substrate-like form of PAI-1. The conversion of the inhibitor to a substrate like form is caused by a conformational change without alteration of the amino acid sequence and is of interest in order to study the mechanism of the interaction between serine protease and SERPIN. In this manuscript we demonstrate the cleavage of PAI-1 and discuss the possible mechanism by which a SERPIN is cleaved by its target protease.

CHARACTERISTICS OF PAI-1

Tissue type plasminogen activator (tPA) and urokinase type plasminogen activator (uPA) are serine proteases which activates plasminogen to the active enzyme plasmin, which is an initial step of fibrinolysis[11]. PAI-1 is a member of the SERPIN family and inhibits uPA and both single chain type- and two chain-type tPA[12-14]. In plasma the activity of PAs, therefore, are primarily controlled by the balance of PAs and PAI-1. The physiological relevance of PAI-1 is proved by the facts that the plasma levels of PAI-1 inversely correlates with fibrinolytic activity both in the plasma and in the euglobulin fraction[15].

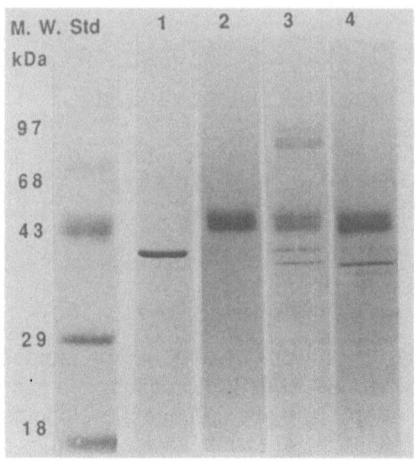 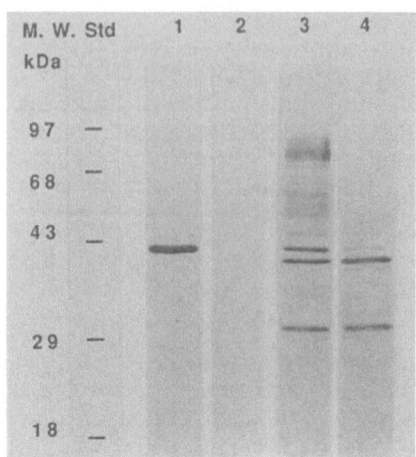

Fig. 1. The cleavage of rpPAI-1 by uPA after SDS treatment.

Samples of active rpPAI-1 (lane 1) was preincubated with saline (lane 3) or 0.1% SDS (lane 4) for 20 min. at room temperature followed by the addition of 1.0% Triton X-100. Samples were then incubated with uPA (shown in lane 2) for 30 minutes at 37°C before analyzed by SDS-PAGE under non-reducing condition. Protein bands were stained either with Coomassie Brilliant Blue (A: left) or with immuno blot analysis (B: right).

Most of eukaryotic PAI-1 obtained from conditioned medium of endothelial cell culture are reported to be in an inactive form that can be subsequently activated by denaturants such as SDS or guanidine hydrochloride (guanidine HCl)[16]. The inactive form of PAI-1 is denoted latent PAI-1[14]. In the present study we employed recombinant prokaryotic PAI-1 (rpPAI-1) expressed by E. Coli. Most of rpPAI-1 was found to be in an inherently active form and its activity was not increased even after guanidine HCl treatment[17]. rpPAI-1 is not glycosylated and therefore has a molecular weight slightly smaller than that of eukaryotic PAI-1, but kinetic' characteristics of rpPAI-1 are essentially the same as those of either active or guanidine HCl activated human recombinant eukaryotic PAI-1 (rePAI-1)[17]. We employed this inherently active rpPAI-1 and studied the effects of SDS on both the function and the conformation. We then discovered that in the presence of 0.1% SDS rpPAI-1 was cleaved at the reactive center by PAs[10].

CLEAVAGE OF PAI-1 BY PAS.

Most of rpPAI-1 employed in the present study had an inherent inhibitory activity and forms a complexes with both uPA and tPA. However, when this material was pretreated with 0.01% SDS and was neutralized with 1.0% Triton X-100, it lost its inhibitory activity and did not form complexes with PAs. Moreover when it was pretreated by 0.1% SDS and was neutralized with 1.0%

Triton X-100, it was cleaved by PAs to smaller molecular weight forms (Fig. 1). Amino acid sequence analysis of cleaved PAI-1 revealed that it was cleaved at its reactive center[10]. The cleaved form of rpPAI-1 was inactive and did not form complexes with PAs.

Since rpPAI-1 which was pretreated by 0.1% SDS was easily cleaved by PAs, we defined this form as "substrate-like form". This form has little activity to inhibit the amidolytic activity of PAs[10], which fits its inability to form a stoichiometric complex with PAs. Including the substrate-like form, PAI-1 may adopt three different forms. The first is the active form, the second is the latent form and the third is the substrate-like form. Although both the latent and substrate forms of PAI-1 are found in conditioned medium of cultured eukaryotic cells, it is controversial whether these forms of PAI-1 exists in plasma milieu.

THE CONFORMATION OF SUBSTRATE-LIKE FORM OF PAI-1.

As determined by circular dichroism analysis the substrate-like form of PAI-1 obtained by SDS treatment has a different conformation from both its active form and latent form[10]. The CD spectra of active PAI-1 in the absence of SDS showed broad negative band in the range of wavelength from 205 to 250 nm with the maximum magnitude of about -1.7 at 220 nm. This rather small magnitude of the spectra suggests that it contains a lower content of α-helices. A calculation of the content of α-helices by elipiticity at 208 nm revealed an α-helical content of less than 1.0 %. Treatment with 0.1 % SDS decreased the negative signal and showed double minimum pattern (208 and 222 nm), which indicates that the content of α-helices was significantly increased. Calculations by elipiticity at 208 nm revealed an α-helical content of 27.9 % at 0.1 % SDS. The increase of the α-helical content by SDS treatment allowed us to calculate structural elements further by spectral resolution technique. PAI-1 treated with 0.1 % SDS contained Helices 37%, Beta 28%, Turn 17% and Random 19%. These results are comparable to the 40% of pleated sheet and 39% of α-helices, which were observed by X-ray crystallography of the reactive site cleaved form of α1-antitrypsin(α1AT)[4]. This enzymatically cleaved form of α1AT obviously has a different conformation from its native form[4], in which P1 and P1' residues are split to the far opposite sites and the peptide loop is inserted to the middle of the molecule. It is interesting that the substrate-like form without the cleavage adopt the similar conformation to the reactive site cleaved SERPIN.

CLEAVAGE OF OTHER SERPINS BY THEIR SPECIFIC SERINE PROTEASES.

The cleavage of other SERPINS by their target proteases have also been reported. Carrel et. al.[18] employed a peptide annealing technique and succeeded to obtain a modified form of antithrombin-III (ATIII). By mixing intact ATIII and the peptides corresponding to either the P7-P14 or the P2-P14 region of the reactive bond loop of ATIII, they obtained structural changes of ATIII from a stressed form to a new stable locked conformation and a relaxed form which is similar to the cleaved form of ATIII, respectively. Björk et. al.[19] also employed the similar technique and reported that the binding of a tetradecapeptide corresponding to the P1 to P14 of ATIII to an ATIII molecule altered both the function and the conformation of ATIII. They proved that the peptide bound ATIII did not form a complex with thrombin but was cleaved at its reactive center by its target protease thrombin. Both groups showed that the conformation of peptide (P2-P14 or P1-P14) bound ATIII is similar to the reactive bond cleaved ATIII. From these data and the analysis of the crystal structure of cleaved α1-AT, Carrel et. al. concluded that the insertion of the peptide loop to the middle of the molecule by either the cleavage of the reactive center or the annealing of the synthesized peptide of reactive bond loop, result in the conversion of the native stressed form to the relaxed form[18]. Moreover, the insertion of the peptides by annealing technique facilitate the interaction between exposed loop of SERPIN and the active site of protease and also prevents the insertion of the cleaved peptide loop to the middle of the molecule, which results in the reduction of the trapping ability of the enzyme since the partial insertion of the reactive bond loop is suggested to play an important role to trap the enzyme[19,20].

As studied by circular dichroism the conformational alteration of ATIII from the native stressed form to the relaxed form[18] is very similar to our data on PAI-1 in which conformational transformation was obtained by SDS treatment. In both cases, the magnitude of the negative band in the spectral region below 230 nm increased and two minima appeared at 208 nm and 220 nm, which indicates a significant increase of α-helical structures. It is therefore possible that SDS treatment introduces the conformation in which strained loop is interrupted from being inserted to the middle of the molecule as shown by a peptide annealing technique. In such case the contents of α-helix is larger probably due to a helical conformation of an exposed reactive center. These data also agree to the hypothesis that mobile reactive center is necessary for the inhibitory activity.

CONGENITALLY ABNORMAL SUBSTRATE-LIKE SERPINS

Congenitally abnormal substrate-like form of SERPINS have been reported. α2-antiplasmin(α2AP) Enschede is a variant of α2AP associated with serious bleeding tendency[21]. Analyses of the amino acid sequence of purified α2-AP Enschede revealed that an alanine was inserted supplementary between p9-p10 in normal α2AP and the reactive center was moved downstream by a space of an amino acid[21]. α2-AP Enschede does not form a stoichiometric complex with plasmin but is cleaved at the reactive center by plasmin as it were a substrate of plasmin[22]. ATIII Hamilton[23] and ATIII Glasgow II[24] are variants of ATIII, which defect reactivity against serine proteases. It lacks the activity to form a complex with thrombin either in the presence or absence of Heparin but

Table 1 **Substrate-Like Abnormal SERPIN**

	abnormality	symptom
ATIII-Hamilton a) ATIII-Glasgow II b)	substitution P12 Ala to Thr	thrombosis
C1 inhibitor Ma c)	substitution P12 Ala to Glu	angioedema
α2-AP Enschede d)	insertion of Ala between P9 and P10	bleeding

a)[22,23]   b)[24]   c)[20]   d)[21]

was cleaved by both thrombin and factor Xa.   Purified ATIII Hamilton revealed that P12 Ala was substituted by Thr.   C1 inhibitor Ma, in which P12 Ala is substituted by Glu, is also a substrate form of SERPIN and is cleaved by plasma kallikrein[20].   It was suggested that the sequence at the position between P10 and P14 are rather conserved in the active SERPINS and that non inhibitory SERPINS like ovoalubumin or angiotensinogen has different sequence in this region[18,25].   These three substrate-like abnormal SERPINS also have abnormalities in this region, which support the suggestion that P10-P14 plays an important role for the mobility of the reactive center that may be essential for the inhibitory activity.   In these abnormal SERPINS the reactive center is most likely interfered to be inserted to the middle of the protein and exposed helical reactive site is easily cleaved by their target proteases.

REFERENCES

1. Doolittle RF (1983)   Science 222: 417-419.

2. Carrel RW and Boswell DR (1986) In: A. Barret and G. Salvensen (eds) Proteinase inhibitors. Elsevier. Amsterdam. pp. 403-420

3. Carrell RW, Pemberton PA and Boswell DR (1987)   Cold Spring Harb Symp Quant Biol 52: 527-35.

4. Loebermann H, Tokuoka R, Deisenhofer J and Huber R (1984)   J Mol Biol 177: 531-556.

5. Huber R and Carrell RW (1989)   Biochemistry 28: 8951-66.

6. Matheson NR, van HH and Travis J (1991)   J Biol Chem 266: 13489-91.

7. Shieh BH, Potempa J and Travis J (1989)   J Biol Chem 264: 13420-3.

8. Lawrence DA, Strandberg L, Ericson J and Ny T (1990)   J Biol Chem 265: 20293-301.

9. Lindahl TL, Ohlsson PI and Wiman B (1990)   Biochem J 265: 109-13.

10. Urano T, Strandberg L, Johansson LB-Å and Ny T (in press)   Eur J Biochem

11. Castellino FJ (1981)   Chem Rev 81: 431-446.

12. Loskutoff DJ, van MJ, Erickson LA and Lawrence D (1983)   Proc Natl Acad Sci U S A 80: 2956-60.

13. Ny T, Sawdey M, Lawrence D, Millan JL and Loskutoff DJ (1986)   Proc Natl Acad Sci U S A 83: 6776-80.

14. Loskutoff DJ, Sawdey M and Mimuro J (1989)   Prog Hemost Thromb 9: 87-115.

15. Urano T, Sakakibara K, Rydzewski A, Urano S, Takada Y and Takada A (1990) Thromb Haemost 63: 82-6.

16. Hekman CM and Loskutoff DJ (1985)   J Biol Chem 260: 11581-7.

17. Lawrence D, Strandberg L, Grundstrom T and Ny T (1989)   Eur J Biochem 186: 523-33.

18. Carrell RW, Evans DL and Stein PE (1991)   Nature 353: 576-8.

19. Björk I, Ylinenjärvi K, Olson ST and Bock PE (1992)   J Biol Chem 25: 1976-1982.

20. Skriver K, Wikoff WR, Patston PA, Tausk F, Schapira M, Kaplan AP and Bock SC (1991)   J Biol Chem 266: 9216-21.

21. Holmes WE, Lijnen HR, Nelles L, Kluft C, Nieuwenhuis HK, Rijken DC and Collen D (1987)   Science 238: 209-11.

22. Rijken DC, Groeneveld E, Kluft C and Nieuwenhuis HK (1988)   Biochem J 255: 609-15.

23. Austin RC, Rachubinski RA, Ofosu FA and Blajchman MA (1991)   Blood 77: 2185-2189.

24. Ireland H, Lane DA, Thompson E, Walker ID, Blench I, Morris HR, Freyssinet JM, Grunebaum L, Olds R and Thein SL (1991)   Br J Haematol 79: 70-4.

25. Perry DJ, Harper PL, Fairham S, Daly M and R.W. C (1989)   FEBS Lett 254: 174-176.

THE STRUCTURAL CHARACTERIZATION OF COAGULATION FACTOR IX/FACTOR X-BINDING PROTEIN ISOLATED FROM THE VENOM OF *TRIMERESURUS FLAVOVIRIDIS*

TAKASHI MORITA AND HIDEKO ATODA

Department of Biochemistry, Meiji College of Pharmacy, Tokyo, Japan

INTRODUCTION

Inhibitor of the activation of prothrombin have been found in the venoms of *Agkistrodon acutus* (1) and *Trimeresurus gramineus* (2). The anticoagulant isolated from *A. acutus* inhibited the participation of factor Xa in the prothrombinase complex (3). Teng and Seegers have also reported that the activation of prothrombin was inhibited by a protein from *A. acutus* venom through its binding to factor Xa (4). We have developed a simple procedure of affinity chromatography on a column of insoluble factor X-Cellulofine to detect and concomitantly to isolate the factor X-binding protein from the venom of *Deinagkistrodon acutus*. We indicated that one of the anticoagulants in the venom of *D. acutus* is a factor X-binding protein.

During initial screening of factor X-binding proteins in various snake venoms by means of affinity chromatography on a column of factor X-Cellulofine, we found that the venom of *T. flavoviridis* (Habu snake) contained a high level of a factor X-binding protein with anticoagulant activity. In addition, the anticoagulant was found to bind not only to factor X as well as factor Xa, but also to factor IX as well as to factor IXa (5). In this paper we describe the isolation, characterization, and the entire amino acid sequence of the anticoagulant protein with factor IX/factor X-binding ability from the venom of *T. flavoviridis*. In the present study, we also determined the pattern of disulfide bonds in IX/X-bp. Information on the pattern of disulfide bonds in the anticoagulant protein, together with results of crystallographic studies (6) could provide further information about the function of IX/X-bp.

MATERIALS AND METHODS

Lysyl endopeptidase from *Achromobactor lyticus* M497-1 was obtained from Wako Pure Chemicals Industries, Tokyo. α-Chymotrypsin treated with TLCK was obtained from Sigma Chemical Co., St. Louis. The Cosmosil $5C_{18}$ column (5 mm i. d. x 150 mm) and the Finepak SIL $C_{18}S$ column (4.6 mm i. d. x 150 mm) were obtained from Nacalai Tesque, Inc. Kyoto, and Japan Spectroscopic Co., Ltd., Tokyo, respectively. Amino acid analysis was performed as previously described (7). Cystine-contain-

35

ing peptides, identified by amino acid analysis, were subjected to automated sequence analysis with a model 473A protein sequencer from Applied Biosystems.

RESULTS

A factor X-binding protein with $\underline{M_r}$ = 27,000 was purified from crude venom by S-Sepharose Fast Flow ion-exchange chromatography, as shown in Fig.1. In the experiment presented here, 1.9 mg of anticoagulant protein was obtained from 50 mg of *T. flavoviridis* venom. The anticoagulant protein, factor IX/factor X-binding protein (IX/X-bp) bound with factor IX and factor X in the presence of Ca^{2+} with stoichiometry of 1 to 1.

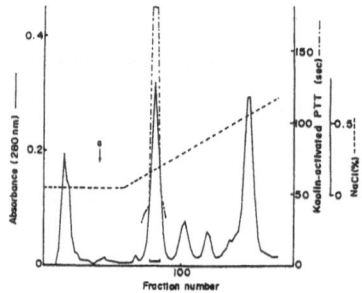

Fig. 1. Column chromatography of venom from *T. flavoviridis* on S-Sepharose Fast Flow.

Analysis of S-pyridylethylated IX/X-bp by sodium dodecyl sulfate-polyacrylamide gel electrophoresis revealed a 16.0 kDa band (designated A chain) and a 15.5 kDa band (designated B chain). These two chains were separated by reversed-phase HPLC and their complete amino acid sequences were deter- mined by sequencing the peptides obtained by digestion with lysyl endopeptidase, chymotrypsin, or *S. aureus* V8 protease and chemical cleavage with cyanogen bromide. The A chain had the amino-termi- nal sequence of Asp-Cys-Leu-Ser-Gly- and consisted of 129 residues with a $\underline{M_r}$ of 14,830, and B chain had the sequence of Asp-Cys-Pro-Ser-Asp- and consisted of 123 residues with a $\underline{M_r}$ of 14,440. There was 47% homology between A chain and B chain (Fig. 2).

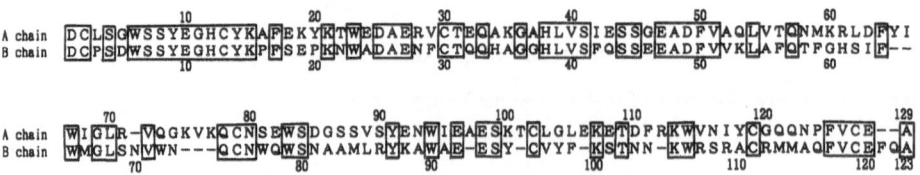

Fig. 2. Alignment of the amino acid sequence of the A and B chains of IX/X-bp.

The sequence of IX/X-bp showed 25-37% homology with that of the C-type carbohydrate recognition domain-like structure of acorn barnacle lectin, human and rat asialoglycoprotein receptors, human lymphocyte Fcε receptor for IgE, proteoglycan core protein, pancreatic stone protein, and tetranectin. Homology with other proteins such as botrocetin, light chain of RVV-X, and galactose-specific lectin, isolated from Crotalidae snake venoms was also observed. The sequences of the first 10 amino acid residues of both chains also had homology with the partial amino acid sequence of the anticoagulant protein (*acutus* factor IX/X-bp) isolated from the venom of *Deinagkistrodon acutus* (Fig. 3).

```
                               1      5        10
Habu IX/X-bp,  A chain        D C L  S G W S S Y E -
Acutus IX/X-bp 1,  A chain    D C P  S G W S S Y E -
Botrocetin,  α chain          D C P  S G W S S Y E -
RVV-X,  L chain          V L  D C P  S G W L S Y E -

                               1      5        10
Habu IX/X-bp,  B chain        D C P  S D W S S Y E -
Acutus IX/X-bp 1,  B chain    D C P  S D W S S Y E -
Botrocetin,  β chain          D C P  P D W S S Y E -
RVV-X,  L chain          V L  D C P  S G W L S Y E -
```

Fig. 3. Sequence homologies between the amino-terminal sequence of IX/X-bps and those of other two-chain, C-type lectin-like proteins from various snake venoms.

The amino acid composition and amino acid sequence of cystine-containing peptides, derived by enzymatic digestion of CNBr-generated fragments of IX/X-bp, were analyzed to determine the location of the seven disulfide bridges in the protein. Three disulfide bridges in the A chain link Cys^2 to Cys^{13}, Cys^{30} to Cys^{127}, and Cys^{102} to Cys^{119}. Three disulfide bridges in the B chain link Cys^2 to Cys^{13}, Cys^{30} to Cys^{119}, and Cys^{96} to Cys^{111}. An interchain disulfide bond links Cys^{79} of the A chain and Cys^{75} of the B chain. The intrachain disulfide-bonding patterns of both the A and B chains of IX/X-bp are similar to those found in other C-type lectin-like proteins.

DISCUSSIONS

The location of seven disulfide bridges are shown in Fig. 4. IX/X-bp is a heterogeneous two-chain protein containing six intrachain disulfide bonds and an interchain disulfide bond.

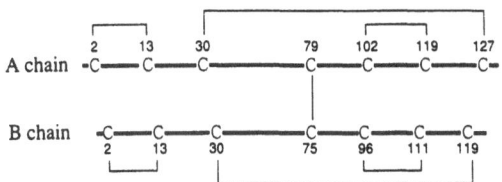

Fig. 4. Schematic representation of IX/X-bp, showing the location of the six intrachain disulfide bridges and the single interchain disulfide bridge.

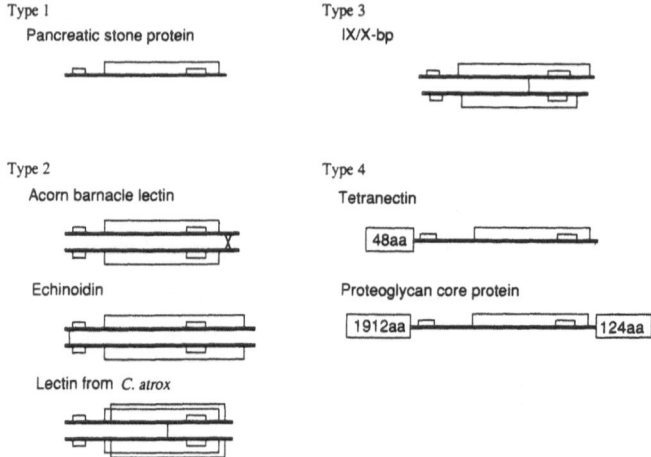

Fig. 5. Disulfide-bonding patterns of C-type lectin-like proteins.
aa, amino acid residues.

There are six proteins containing C-type lectin-like domain of which the primary structure and the pattern of disulfide bridges have been determined to date. Figure 5 shows the disulfide-bonding patterns of IX/X-bp and six other C-type lectin-like domains from, respectively, pancreatic stone protein (8), acorn barnacle lectin (9), echinoidin (10), galactose-specific lectin from *Crotalus atrox* (rattlesnake) venom (11), tetranectin (12), and proteoglycan core protein (13). All these domains share key structural features, including the presence of a small loop at the amino-terminal region and another small loop within a large loop in the carboxy-terminal region. Intrachain disulfide-bonding patterns of both the A and the B chains of IX/X-bp are similar to those of C-type lectin-like domains, indicating that IX/X-bp consists of two covalently linked, heterogeneous, C-type lectin-like subunits. The chain structures of proteins that include C-type lectin-like domains can be classified into four types. First, pancreatic stone protein has a single C-type lectin-like domain. Second, there are covalently linked two-chain proteins which consist of two homogeneous C-type lectin-like subunits, such as acorn barnacle lectin, echinoidin, and the lectin from *C. atrox*. As shown in Figure 5, the locations of inter-chain disulfide bridges in these proteins are different . IX/X-bp is a third type of protein and consists of two heterogeneous subunits. There is also a fourth type of protein, exemplified by proteoglycan core protein and tetranectin, and these proteins contain distinct functional group(s) in addition to C-type lectin-like subunits.

Recently, it was reported that NH$_2$-terminal sequences of the heterodimeric form of botrocetin exhibit an apparent homology to the NH$_2$-terminal regions of C-type lectins (14) (Fig. 3). Botrocetin is a von

Willebrand factor-dependent platelet coaggulutinin, which was isolated from the venom of *Bothrops jararaca* (15). In addition, the sequences have been reported of several proteins with C-type lectin-like structures that have been isolated from the venom of Crotalidae snake, such as the galactose-specific lectin from the venom of *C. atrox* (11), and a light chain of coagulation factor X-activating enzyme (RVV-X) from the venom of *Vipera russelli* (Russell's viper) (16). The extent of the similarily of the amino-terminal thirty-amino-acid sequences between the α chain of botrocetin and the A chain of IX/X-bp is 67% and that between the β chain of botrocetin (14) and the B chain of IX/X-bp is 70%. The extent of the similarity between the A chain of IX/X-bp and the RVV-X light chain and between the A chain and *C. atrox* lectin is 43% and 28%, respectively. The B chain of IX/X-bp and the RVV-X light chain are 48% homologous and *C. atrox* lectin and the B chain are 28% homologous. It is interesting that these structurally related proteins, which probably evolved from a common ancestral protein, have a variety of functions that differ from one another.

IX/X-bp forms a complex with factor X with a molar ratio of 1 to 1 (5). Further investigations are required to determine which subunit of IX/X-bp binds the coagulation factor and whether both subunits of IX/X-bp are necessary for the formation of the complex with the coagulation factor.

We thank Naomitsu Eguchi of Meiji College of Pharmacy for performing amino acid analysis.

REFERENCES

1. Ouyang, C. & Teng, C. M. (1972) *Biochim. Biophys. Acta* **278**, 155-162

2. Ouyang, C. & Yang, F. Y. (1975) *Biochim. Biophys. Acta* **386**, 479-492

3. Ouyang, C. & Teng, C. M. (1973) *Toxicon* **11**, 287-292

4. Teng, C. M. & Seegers, W. H. (1981) *Thromb. Res.* **23**, 255-263

5. Atoda, H. & Morita, T. (1989) *J. Biochem.* **106**, 808-813

6. Mizuno, H., Atoda, H., & Morita, T. (1991) *J. Mol. Biol.* **220**, 225-226

7. Atoda, H., Hyuga, M., & Morita, T. (1991) *J. Biol. Chem.* **266**, 14903-14911

8. Rouimi, P., De Caro, J., Bonicel, J., Rovery, M., & De Caro, A. (1988) *FEBS Lett.* **229**, 171-174

9. Muramoto, K. & Kamiya, H. (1990) *Biochim. Biophys. Acta* **1039**, 52-60

10. Giga, Y., Ikai, A., & Takahashi, K. (1987) *J. Biol. Chem.* **262**, 6197-6203

11. Hirabayashi, J., Kusunoki, T., & Kasai, K. (1991) *J. Biol. Chem.* **266**, 2320-2326

12. Fuhlendorff, J., Clemmensen, I., & Magnusson, S. (1987) *Biochemistry* **26**, 6757-6764

13. Sandy, J. D., Flannery, C. R., Boynton, R. E., & Neame, P. J. (1990) *J. Biol. Chem.* **265**, 21108-21113

14. Fujimura, Y., Titani, K., Usami, Y., Suzuki, M., Oyama, T., Matsui, T., Fukui, H., Sugimoto, M., & Ruggeri, Z. M. (1991) *Biochemistry* **30**, 1957-1964

15. Brinkhous, K. M., Read, M. S., Fricke, W. A., & Wagner, R. H. (1983) *Proc. Natl. Acad. Sci. USA* **80**, 1463-1466

16. Takeya, H., Nishida, S., Miyata, T., Kawada, S., Saisaka, Y., Morita, T., & Iwanaga, S. (1992) *J. Biol. Chem.* **267**, 14109-14117

THE HEMOLYMPH COAGULATION SYSTEM OF SHRIMPS

Inn-Ho Tsai, Yuh-Ling Chen, Ling-Rong Kao, and *Jin-Hua Cheng

Institute of Biological Chemistry, Academia Sinica, Taipei, and
*Tungkang Marine Laboratory, Taiwan Fisheries Res. Inst., Taiwan.

KEY WORDS: Coagulation, Clottable protein, Transglutaminase, (Shrimp)

ABSTRACT

The effects of different anticoagulants on the shrimp coagulation systems were studied. Metal ion chelators, Zn^{2+}, Hg^{2+}, serine protease inhibitors and some transglutaminase-inhibitors were found to inhibit the coagulation. We have purified the clottable proteins (CP) from the hemolymph of marine shrimps *Penaeus monodon* and *Penaeus japonicus* by DEAE-ion exchanger and gel-filtration. The purified CP was cross-linked to form an insoluble clot *in vitro* by the shrimp hemocyte transglutaminase (TG) in the presence of 10^{-4} M Ca^{2+}. Being a dimer of 92 kDa subunits, the shrimp TG is homologous to Factor XIIIa of the mammalian coagulation system, but very unstable especially in presence of Ca^{2+}. The soluble CP-dimers or oligomers are composed of glycoprotein subunits of 180 kDa, which contain 24% glucose and 9% N-acetylglucosamine. Its N-terminal amino acid sequence up to the 25th residue is LQPGLEYQYRYSARVASGIPSINRQ, bearing 72 and 28% similarity to the lobster CP and the *C. elegans* vitellogenin, respectively. Using the rabbit antiserum raised against the shrimp CP for western-blot analysis we found that the CP was present only in the hemolymph and hemopoietic nodule tissue but not in the midgut or the muscle of the shrimp. The rocket immunoelectrophoretic analyses showed specific changes of the hemolymph CP-concentration under different physiological conditions. The anti-CP antiserum also precipitated the CP's in hemolymphs of other penaeid and metapenaeid shrimps but not those of lobster, fresh water prawn (*Macrobrachium rosenbergii*) or marine crab.

INTRODUCTION

The invertebrate model of plasma coagulation may render some messages to modern biology and help us to understand more about the general principles of haemostasis in animals. Crustacean decapods such as lobsters, have been known to have an extracellular protein circulating in the hemolymph that clots *in vivo* under various conditions of trauma, and gels *in vitro* upon the addition of hemocyte lysate or tissue

41

extracts [1]. Early studies also showed that the Crustacean coagulation systems varied from species to species and were classified into three types of different degrees of apparent clotting [2]. From the shrimp hemolymph, at least two kinds of cells (hemocytes) were identified, they differed histochemically and played different role of either coagulating or endocytotic [3,4]. Although the mechanisms of coagulation in lobster, crayfish [5,6] and shrimp [7] have been studied, we know very little about the biochemistry of hemolymph components and the regulation of coagulation in decapods.

In many areas of the world including Taiwan, shrimp aquaculture is economically important; it becomes essential to know the basic biology relating to the production and the disease-control of some important shrimp species. In this paper, we report the results of biochemical studies on the hemolymph coagulation system of two shrimp species, *Penaeus monodon* and *Penaeus japonicus*. Their transglutaminases (TG) and clottable proteins (CP) were purified and characterized.

MATERIALS AND METHODS

Anticoagulant and hemolymph samples Penaeid shrimps in intermolt stage were obtained from fish merchants. Blood samples were withdrawn between the first and second pairs of swimming-legs of shrimp using a 23-gauge needle attached to a 3 ml sterile plastic syringe containing various anticoagulant in isotonic buffer [8]. The region of shrimp shell punctured was first sterilized with 70% alcohol, and care was taken to avoid any contamination from the sea water or generation of air-bubbles in the plasma. The withdrawn plasma (100-800 μl) was centrifuged at 2500 rpm for 10 min at 2-4°C to collect the hemocytes.

Determination of protein Quantitation of protein was carried out by the dye-binding method of Bradford [10] using BSA to establish the standard curve.

Assay and purification of TG Shrimp TG was assay with the system of dansyl cadaverine plus succinyl-casein [11]. The increase of fluorence due to the incorporation of the primary amine into the protein hydrophobic enterior was followed. The shrimp hemocytes were lysed with hypotonic buffer containing EDTA. The transglutaminase was isolated from the hemocyte lysate by Fractogel TSK DEAE-650 (M) and Sephacryl S-300 chromatographies as described previously [12].

Purification of CP After removal of the cell by low-speed

centrifugation, the plasma was dialyzed against 3 l of TE buffer (50 mM Tris-HCl, 1 mM EDTA, pH 8.0), and chromatographed on a TSK DEAE-650 column (2x9 cm) pre-equilibrated in the same TE buffer. The proteins were fractionated by a linear gradient of 0-0.4 N NaCl in the buffer and tested for clottability by the hemocyte lysate. The CP fractions were pooled and lyophilized, then purified with a Sepharose CL-6B column (1.5x100 cm) in TE buffer. Further purification of the CP was effected by HPLC gel filtration through a Zorbax GF-450 column (Du Pont Co.) in 0.2 N ammonium acetate (pH 8.0) [9].

Electrophoresis SDS-polyacrylamide gel electrophoresis was carried out to determine the subunit molecular mass of the CP and the TG using 5% acrylamide, or 3.5% acrylamide plus 0.5% agarose according to the method of Neville [13].

Sequence and carbohydrate determination The N-terminal amino acid of the purified CP was analysed by automated protein sequencing by an Applied Biosystems sequencer (model 477A). Sugar content of the CP was analyzed with a Dionex anion-exchange-chromatography system and the separated sugars were analyzed with a pulsed amperametric detector calibrated with the sugar standards [14].

Antiserum and immunological analysis Purified CP (~300 mg) were collected from the SDS-PAGE gel and used as the antigen to raise rabbit antibody against the shrimp CP. After 2 months of consecutive immunization, high titer (1/1000) antiserum was obtained. Rocket immunoelectrophoresis was performed with 0.85% agarose in 18 mM barbitate buffer (pH 8.6) containing 3% (v/v) of antiserum. The gel was coated 0.2 cm thick on Gel-fix film (Serva Co., Heidelberg) and electrophoresis was run at 100 mV for 3 h after the addition of samples into the wells, as described [15].

RESULT AND DISCUSSION

We have first checked the effects of various anticoagulants on the shrimp coagulation. Heparin, antithrombin III and hirudin could not prevent the plasma from coagulating, but leupeptin and 4-amidino-phenylmethanesulfonyl fluoride (Boehringer Mannheim Co.) did inhibit the coagulation. Chelating agent EDTA, heavy metal ions (Hg^{2+}, Sr^{2+} and Zn^{2+}) and inhibitors for the cross-linking enzyme (e.g. Gly-Gly ethyl ester) are effective anticoagulant. However, the clotting time and the susceptibility toward each anticoagulant varied with respect to the species, e.g. in vitro coagulation in P. japonicus was faster than that of *P. monodon*, and some anticoagulants only prolonged coagulation in the latter but not in the former.

The shrimp plasma is transparent and blue-greyish because of the high content of Cu^{2+}-containing hemocyanin. The volumn of hemocyte pelleted by low speed centrifugation is usually only 1% of that of the plasma. The shrimp TG was purified from the hemocyte lysate of *P. monodon* by ion-exchange and gel-filtration chromatographies. The enzyme activity was measured kinetically either by the *in vitro* clotting time or by the fluorescence enhancement due to the cross-linking of dansyl-cadaverine and succinyl-casein. No initial latent phase in the assay of shrimp TG was observed as in the case of mammalian Factor XIII, nor the addition of any protease was required to activate the shrimp TG. The native molecular mass of the shrimp TG was determined by Sepharose S-300 column to be 184 kDa. Its subunit molecular mass was estimated to be 92 kDa by SDS-PAGE. Thus the shrimp TG was a dimer. Presumably, the shrimp TG was similar to mammalian FXIIIa, but the corresponding b subunits were not found in the shrimp. Partial amino acid sequencing of the CNBr-fragments of shrimp TG purified by HPLC also showed about 50% similarity to the corresponding sequence of the mammalian Factor XIIIa. The TG activity depended on the presence of 0.1-1 mM of Ca^{2+}; and Sr^{2+}, Ba^{2+}, Mg^{2+} and Tb^{3+} could not substitute for Ca^{2+}. However, the activity of the shrimp TG appeared to be transient since in the presence of mM $CaCl_2$ the activity was auto-inactivated in minutes. Antioxidants or reducing agents could only slightly protect, but EDTA could halt this inactivation process. Thus, the enzyme could be stored at 0-2°C with EDTA in buffers of pH 7-8.5 before adding Ca^{2+} for activation.

N-terminal sequences of the 170 and 180 kDa monomers or oligomers of the *P. monodon* CP were found to be similar or identical. The first 25 amino acid residues are LQPGLEYQYRYSARVASGIPSINRQ, which is 72 and 28% identical to the CP from lobster and the vitellogenin from *C. elegans*, respectively [1]. The carbohydrate content of the shrimp CP was analyzed [14] to be mainly 24% glucose, 9% N-acetylglucosamine.

Rabbit antiserum raised against *P. monodon* CP was very useful in the quantitation of CP in the shrimp plasma. The sensitivity of rocket immunoelectrophoresis allow accurate determination of the CP with as low as 0.1 μl of the shrimp hemolymph. The shrimp CP concentrations were in the range of 2-14 mg/ml and appeared to vary with seasons and molt-stages: the concentration is higher in summer than in winter, and increased just before molting. The CP seemed inducible and increased several folds by consecutive withdrawing of the blood, or under trauma conditions.

Ouchterlony double-diffusion tests confirmed that the *P. monodon* CP was immunochemically related to the CP's from other penaeid and metapenaeid species but not those of the spiny lobster, marine crab or fresh water prawn (*Macrobrachium rosenbergii*). The antiserum also was used in a western-blot analysis to locate the CP in the tissues of *P. monodon*. It was found that only the hemopoietic nodule and the hemolymph contained the protein but not the midgut or the muscle of the shrimp.

ACKNOWLEDGEMENTS
This work was supported by research grants of the National Science Council and Council of Agriculture of the Republic of China. We thank Dr. C. S. Liu for the carbohydrate analysis of CP.

REFERENCE
[1] Doolittle RF, Riley M (1990) Biochem Biophys Res Comm 167: 16-19
[2] Tait J (1911) J Marin Biol Assoc UK 9: 191-198
[3] Hose JE, Martin GG, Gerard AS (1990) Biol Bull 178: 33-45
[4] Omori SA, Martin GG, Hose JE (1989) Cell Tissue Res 255: 117-123
[5] Durliat M (1985) Biol Rev 60: 473-498
[6] Durliat M, Vranckx R (1989) Comp Biochem Physiol 92B: 595-603
[7] Martin GG, Hose JE, Omori S, Chong C, Hoodbhoy T, McKrell N (1991) Comp Biochem Physiol 100B: 517-522
[8] Tsai IH, Chen YL, Lu PJ (1991) In: Reports on Fish Disease Res. XI, Kou KH (ed) COA Fisheries Series No.29. Taipei. Taiwan. pp.22-30
[9] Chen YL, Huang SH, Cheng JH, Tsai IH (1993) In: Reports on Fish Disease Res. XIII, Kou KH (ed) COA Fisheries Series. Taipei. Taiwan. (in press)
[10] Bradford M (1976) Anal Biochem 72: 248-254
[11] Lorand L, Conrad SM (1984) Mol Cell Biochem 58: 9-35
[12] Kao LR (1987) Studies on shrimp (*P. monodon*) hemolymph clotting system and its transglutaminase. Master thesis, Taiwan Univ., Taipei
[13] Neville DM Jr (1971) J Biol Chem 246: 6328-6334
[14] Hardy MR, Townsend RR, Lee YC (1988) Anal Biochem 170: 54-60
[15] Laurell CB (1966) Anal Biochem 15: 45-52

Disorders of coagulation, fibrinolysis, platelets and thrombosis

STUDIES OF FACTOR VIII INHIBITORS IN CHINESE HEMOPHILIA A PATIENTS

MING-CHING SHEN, SHU-WHA LIN, PEI-CHU YANG AND CHIN-CHIN HUANG

Department of Laboratory Medicine and Graduate Institute of Medical Technology, College of Medicine, National Taiwan University, Taipei, Taiwan, Republic of China.

INTRODUCTION

It has been recognized that hemophilic patients with clotting factor inhibitors bleed no more frequently and no worse than patients who do not have this complication. However, the management of bleeding in these patients is a major problem. Low responders can be treated effectively with high doses of clotting factor, whereas treatment is difficult when the clotting factor inhibitor titer is high. Therefore, the diagnosis of the presence of clotting factor inhibitor, immunologic characterization of the inhibitor and investigation of the interaction of the inhibitor with clotting factor become very important in the management of the hemophiliacs with inhibitor[1]. Recent advances in the development of gene cloning and expression have made it possible to characterize in detail, the epitopes recognized by inhibitors. This epitope mapping helps us to understand the structure and function relationship of factor VIII protein and also the mechanism by which these factor VIII inhibitors react[2,3]. This paper is to present the immunologic characterization and kinetic studies of factor VIII inhibitors found in six patients and epitope mapping of one of the inhibitors.

MATERIALS AND METHODS

Subjects

A series of 81 cases of hemophilia A seen at the hematologic section of National Taiwan University Hospital (NTUH) during 1979 to 1981 and 151 cases at the hemophilia center of the same NTUH during 1988 to 1990 were studied.

Methods

Factor VIII:C assay was performed according to the one-stage method of Lossing et al[4]. The Bethesda unit, a factor VIII inhibitor unit, was determined according to the method of Kasper et al with a slight modification in which citrate saline was used, instead of imidazole buffer as a diluent[5,6]. Immunologic characterization of the factor VIII inhibitor was done as described by Feinstein et al[7]. The classification of factor VIII inhibitors or antibodies as type I or type II were according to the criteria of Biggs and coworkers[8,9]. The kinetic analysis and factor VIII:C inactivation by antibodies were done as reported previously[10]. The effect of factor VIII inhibitors on thrombin activation of highly purified factor VIII:C (Hemophil M) was studied as follows: equal volumes of one ml of Hemophil M and one ml of diluted inhibitor or one ml of diluting fluid as control were incubated at 37°C for two hours, then factor VIII:C activity was measured before and 10 min, 20 min, 30 min, 40 min and 50 min after addition of five ul of diluted thrombin (5 u/ml).

Approaches to epitope mapping of factor VIII inhibitor[2,3,]

1. Construction of a factor VIII expressing library using lambda ZAP II as a vector.

    1) The factor VIII cDNA libraries were kindly provided by Dr. Darrel Stafford (University of North Carolina, Chapel Hill, NC, USA) and Dr. Jerry Ware (Scripps, San Diego, USA).

    2) Both libraries were inserted into a lambda-ZAP II vector (Stratagene, La Jolla, CA, USA).The constructed lambda phage libraries were then used for screening after amplification.

2. Synthesis of the factor VIII fusion peptides by induction of the promotor activity.

    1) Approximately 1×10^5 phages were mixed with 0.6ml of the XLI-Blue E. coli culture, 7.5ml melted top agarose were added to the mixture and plated on a 150 mm petri dish and incubated at 37°C.

    2) Synthesis of factor VIII fusion peptides were induced by overlaying on the plate a nitrocellulose (NC) paper impregnated with 10mM isopropyl-β-D-thiogalacto-pyranoside (IPTG).

    3) After incubation at 37°C overnight, the NC paper was marked for reference and removed from the plate.

3. Identification of antibody reactive phage clones by immunoscreening with patient's plasma.

    1) Plasma (or serum) was preabsorbed with an aliquot of the E. coli XLI-Blue crude lysates before being incubated with NC papers at 4°C overnight in the presence of TBS-BSA (Tris buffer saline-bovine serum albumin).

    2) The NC papers were subsequently incubated at 4°C for two hours with an aliquot of alkaline phosphatase-conjugated anti-human IgG (H+L) in TBS-BSA and then transferred to the color development solution (NBT, nitroblue tetrazolium, and BCIP, 5-bromo-4-chloro-3-indolyl phosphate).

    3) Positive clones will appear as purple plaques on the white NC papers.

4. Plaque purification to obtain single clones.

    Immunoreactive phages were then isolated and further screened at a lower phage titer several times for purification.

5. DNA sequencing of factor VIII DNA fragments from immunoreactive phage clones by dideoxy chain termination method.

    1) The purified immunoreactive phages were cultured in large quantity after in vivo excision.

    2) The phage DNA was extracted, cleaved with EcoRI, and were subcloned into sequencing vector M13 mp 18[2,11,12].

    3) The DNA sequences of factor VIII inserts were determined by dideoxy chain termination method using ^{35}S-dATP[13].

6. Alignment of the translated amino acid sequence from each factor VIII cDNA insert.

    1) Distinct phages immunoreactive to the inhibitor were isolated and characterized.

    2) An overlapping factor VIII cDNA fragment was deduced from these positive clones.

RESULT

We have tested the presence of inhibitors in 81 cases of hemophilia A in the years of 1979 to 1981 and 151 cases in the years of 1988 to 1990, 9.9% and 10.6% of them have developed inhibitors respectively. Only patients with severe type had inhibitors.

Immunologic characterization of six factor VIII inhibitors by factor VIII neutralization test revealed that all were IgG type antibodies, four of them were κ-type light chain, the other two were both κ and λ-type light chain.

We have studied kinetic analysis and effects of factor VIII inhibitors on thrombin activation of factor VIII:C in six patients. The relationship of residual factor VIII:C activity in logarithmic scale to antibody concentration was determined after a two hour incubation with normal plasma at 37°C. The factor VIII:C inactivation by four antibodies from hemophilia A patients II, III, V and VI fulfills the criteria of so called type I antibodies. In sufficient quantities, the antibody can completely inactivate factor VIII:C with second order kinetics and there is a linear relationship i.e. a simple kinetics, when the logarithm of residual factor VIII:C activity is compared to the antibody concentration. One of the example representing factor VIII:C inactivating by two antibodies from patients II and VI is shown in Fig.1:1.

The factor VIII:C inactivation by two antibodies from a nonhemophilic patient I and a hemophilic patient IV fulfills the criteria of so called type II antibody, it does not completely inactivate factor VIII:C, even in high concentration, and the factor VIII:C inactivation graph had a curvilinear relationship of residual factor VIII:C activity and antibody concentration i.e. a complex kinetics. Factor VIII:C inactivation by the antibody from patient I is shown in Fig. 1:2.

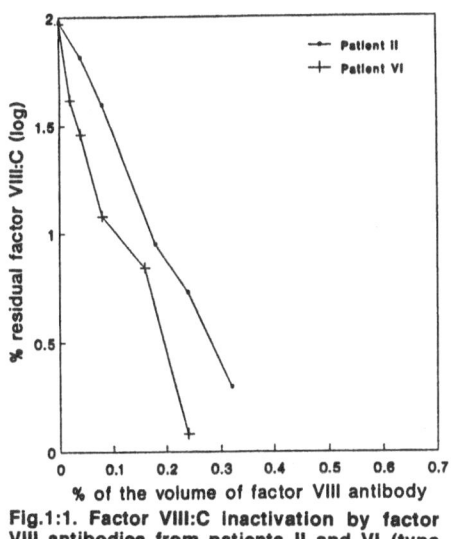

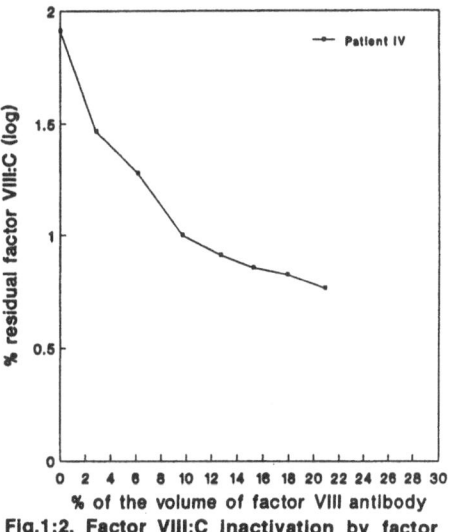

Fig.1:1. Factor VIII:C inactivation by factor VIII antibodies from patients II and VI (type I antibody)

Fig.1:2. Factor VIII:C inactivation by factor VIII antibodies form patient IV (type II antibody)

A fixed volume of normal saline was added to various volumes of patients' plasma to obtain factor VIII antibodies of different concentrations. To the latter, or imidazole buffer as a control, equal volume of normal pool plasma was added. The mixture was incubated at 37°C for two hours then measured for residual factor VIII:C activity, which was expressed as the percent activity of the control and plotted in logarithmic scale.

The basis for nonlinear inactivation by type II antibody was studied by incubating plasma-antibody mixtures with protein-A-Sepharose (PAS) to remove most IgG and any immune complexes formed by IgG1, IgG2, IgG4 antibodies. There was no additional factor VIII:C inactivation when type II antibody from nonhemophilic patient I and plasma mixtures were absorbed with PAS. Thus, the nonlinear and incomplete factor VIII:C inactivating characteristics of type II factor VIII antibody seen when incubated with plasma cannot be attributed to the formation of immune complexes that retain factor VIII:C activity.

The potential role of another factor, i.e. interference by the vonWillebrand factor (VWF), should be also considered. In this study type II factor VIII antibody was tested with purified factor VIII:C, Hemophil M in which there is approximately only one percent of VWF activity. This type II antibody inactivated much more factor VIII:C, i.e. type I property, when it was seperated from VWF protein, and no further augmentation of antibody potency was observed if the antibody-VIII:C mixture was absorbed with PAS. These results suggested that VWF protein inhibited factor VIII:C binding by this type II antibody.

The other type II antibody from hemophilic patient IV had the same type II characteristics when tested with purified factor VIII:C, the pattern was similar to that observed with plasma. However. the adsorption of immune complexes by PAS removed factor VIII:C activity in this case, this indicated that antibody-VIII:C interaction produced an immune complex that retained factor VIII:C activity.

Type I antibody from hemophilic patient II had similar inactivating properties when tested with either purified factor VIII:C or plasma. Subsequent adsorption of the antibody-VIII:C mixture with PAS had no further significant effect on the amount of residual factor VIII:C. Therefore, VWF protein did not affect the VIII:C inactivating property of this type I antibody.

The effect of patients' antibodies on thrombin activation of purified factor VIII:C was studied. Among the factor VIII antibodies studied, one type I antibody from patient II was shown to have no effect on thrombin activation of purified factor VIII:C. The other five antibodies all had inhibitory effect on thrombin activation of purified VIII:C as compared to the control.

In an attempt to localize epitopes recognized by the factor VIII antibodies from these patients, we have tried to map epitopes from the data of kinetic studies and effects of patients' antibodies on thrombin activation of purified factor VIII:C. The results were shown in Fig.2.

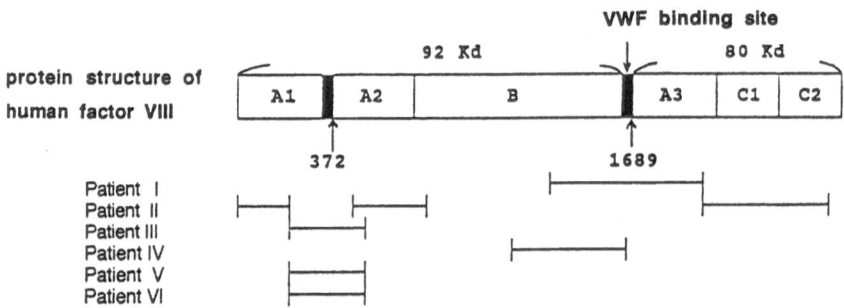

Fig.2. Putative epitopes deduced from kinetic studies and effects on thrombin activation of factor VIII antibodies from six patients. Patient I had type II antibody, the epitope at least included the acidic region, position 1649 to 1689 encompassing the VWF protein binding site. Patient II had type I antibody, the epitopes could be in some region excluding the thrombin cleavage site and VWF protein binding site. Patient III, V and VI all had type I antibody, the epitope at least included the region around position 372, the thrombin cleavage site, and did not include VWF protein binding site. Patient IV had type II antibody, the epitope could be the region including the VWF protein binding site and the position 1689, but not extending further, thus it did not inactivate factor VIII:C completely.

1. Patient I had type II antibody and VWF protein inhibited factor VIII:C binding by this antibody, moreover it affected thrombin activation. The epitopes might include thrombin cleavage sites, positions 372 or 1689. Therefore it at least included the acidic region, position 1649 to 1689, which encompassed the VWF protein binding site.

2. Patient II had type I antibody, the antibody did not affect thrombin activation in vitro. These data suggested that the putative epitopes could be in some region excluding the thrombin cleavage site (positions 372 and 1689) and VWF protein binding site.

3. Patient III, patient V and patient VI all had type I antibody, and the antibody affected thrombin activation, therefore the epitope at least included the region around position 372, the thrombin cleavage site, and did not include VWF protein binding site.

4. Patient IV had type II antibody and the anitbody affected thrombin activation as the type II antibody from patient I, however the antibody did not inactivate purified factor VIII:C completely and their complex retain factor VIII:C activity. These data suggested that the epitope could be the region including the VWF protein binding site and position 1689, the thrombin cleavage site, but not extending further, thus it did not inactivate factor VIII:C completely.

The preliminary data of the putative epitopes recognized by the factor VIII inhibitor of 600 B.U.from patient II was further confirmed by the epitope mapping study. We have plated 10^5 pages per petri dish and screened a total of 5×10^5 phages. The ratio of positive clones was 0.2% in primary screening. Positive clone was about 1.2% in the second screening, and more than 50% in the third screening. Almost pure clones were obtained in the fourth screening. The final procedure was alignment of the translated amino acid sequence from each factor VIII cDNA insert:

1. 32 distinct immunoreactive phages to the inhibitor were isolated and characterized.

2. An overlapping factor VIII cDNA fragment representing.amino acid residues 334-357 was deduced from these 32 positive clones.

DISCUSION

The IgG type of factor VIII inhibitor characterized in the present study of one nonhemophilic case and five hemiophilia A cases is consistent with the previous reports[1,14], whereas both κ and λ type indentified in two antibodies of the five hemophilic inhibitors are unusual as compared to those reported previously, few of hemophilic factor VIII inhibitors have been identified as a mixture of κ and λ type[14].

The epitopes defined in our molecular biological studies, corresponding to amino acid residues 334-357 of the mature factor VIII protein, is encompassing the first activated protein C cleavage site (Arg 336) and locates very close to the thrombin cleavage site (Arg 372), both of which are improtant for biological function of factor VIII[15]. It is conceivable that an antibody recognizing this region might probably inhibit the normal function of factor VIII. The putative epitopes deduced from kinetic studies and the effect of thrombin activation for the same hemophilic factor VIII antibody is consistent with the epitopes defined in the molecular biological studies, a region excluding the thrombin cleavage site as well as the VWF binding site.

One murine anti-factor VIII monoclonal antibody, C5, which inhibit factor VIII:C activity, has been demonstrated to recognize a peptide region of residues 351-365 of factor VIII [16]. A similar epitope, residues 338-362 of factor VIII, has also been identified for a human hemophilic factor VIII inhibitor by analogous approaches[3].

It is our anticipation that specific adsorption of the inhibitors might be achieved by interaction of the inhibitors with antigens which can be factor VIII or regions of factor VIII containing epitopes recognized by these inhibitors. Similar trials have been reproted that a specific immunoadsorption of inhibitors has been successfully performed to remove antibodies in hemophilia B patients[17].

In conclusion, putative epitopes were deduced from kinetic studies and the effect on thrombin activation for six factor VIII inhibitors. For one type I antibody, not interfering to thrombin activation, the epitopes locate conceivably in regions excluding thrombin cleavage site as well as the VWF protein binding site, these preliminary data were further confirmed by molecular biological approaches.

REFERENCES

1. Shen MC (1982) J Formosan Med Assoc 81: 364-379

2. Ware J, Toomey JR, Stafford DW (1988) Proc Natl Acad Sci USA 85: 3165-3169

3. Lubahn BC, Ware J, Staffrod DW, Reisner HM (1989) Blood 73: 497-499

4. Lossing TS, Kasper CK, Feinstein DI (1977) Blood 49: 793-797

5. Kasper CK, Aledort LM, Counts RB, Edson JR, Fratantoni J, Green D, Hampton JW, Hilgartner MW, Lazerson J, Levine PH, McMillan CW, Poul JG, Shapiro SS, Shulman NR, Van Eys J (1975) Thromb Diath Haemorrh 34: 869-872

6. Kasper CK (1975) Thromb Diath Haemorrh 34: 875-876

7. Feinstein DI, Rapaport SI, Chong MNY (1969) Blood 34: 85-90

8. Biggs R, Austen DEG, Denson KWE, Rizza CR, Borrett R (1972) Br J Haematol 23: 125-135

9. Biggs R, Austen DEG, Denson KWE, Borrett R, Rizza CR (1972) Br J Haematol 23: 137-155

10. Gawryl MS, Hoyer LW (1982) Blood 60: 1103-1109

11. Maniatis T, Fritsch EF, Sambrook J (1989) Molecular cloning: a laboratory manual, Cold Spring Harbor Laboratory. Cold spring Habor, New York

12. Messing J (1983) Methods in enzymology 101: 20-89

13. Sanger F, Nichlen S, Coulson AR (1977) Proc Natl Acad Sci USA 74: 5463-5467

14. Hoyer LW, Gawryl MS, Fuente Bdl (1984) In: Hoyer LW (eds) Progress in clinical and biological research volume 150, Factor VIII inhibitors Alan R Liss, Inc New York. pp.73-89

15. White II GC, Shoemaker CB (1989) Blood 73: 1-12

16. Foster PA, Fulcher CA, Houghten RA, Mahoney SDG, Zimmerman TS (1988) J Clin Invest 82: 123-128

17. Nilsson IM, Freiburghaus C, Sundqvist SB, Sandberg H (1984) Plasma Ther Transfus Technol 5:127

HEMOPHILIA A: CHARACTERIZATION OF GENETIC DEFECTS BY THE SINGLE STRAND CONFORMATION POLYMORPHISM (SSCP)

SHU-WHA LIN, SHU-RUNG LIN, AND MING-CHING SHEN.

Graduate Institute of Medical Technology, Hematology Center, and Department of Clinical Pathology, National Taiwan University, School of Medicine, Taipei, Taiwan, ROC.

INTRODUCTION

Hemophilia A is an X-linked hereditary bleeding disorder caused by deleterious mutations in the gene coding for factor VIII. Factor VIII deficiency is heterogeneous and patients are categorized into severe, moderate and mild hemophiliacs according to the levels of their functional factor VIII. Approximately 1/3 of the cases are due to *de novo* mutations[1]. Factor VIII is important for normal hemostasis in that it participates in the intrinsic pathway of the coagulation cascade and serves as a cofactor for factor IX. And it accelerates the enzymatic reaction of the activation of factor X by activated factor IX. The generated factor Xa then activates prothrombin to thrombin which then cleaves fibrinogen to fibrin.

The cDNA and gene coding for human factor VIII have been cloned and characterized[2-5]. The gene is 180 kb in length, containing 26 exons and 25 introns. The amino acid sequence of factor VIII, as deduced from the cDNA sequence, is 2,351 residues long whose primary structure comprises of several domains. The enormous size and heterogeneity of the abnormal factor VIII genes have made it difficult to study the genetic basis in hemophilia A. With the advance of the polymerase chain reaction (PCR), it has been possible to analyze a large and complicated gene like factor VIII. We have tried to elucidate the genetic basis of our hemophilia A patients. Due to the large size and complexity of the factor VIII gene, we decided to use the single-strand conformation polymorphism (SSCP) to search for mutated regions[6,7]. Using SSCP followed by direct sequencing we have identified mutations for 18 patients with hemophilia A. The results we presented here represent a distinct hemophilic population of asian origin.

MATERIALS AND METHODS

Patients All patients were diagnosed as severe, moderate or mild hemophilia with variable amounts of circulating factor VIII measured by the activated partial thromboplastin time (aPTT) as described previously[8].

Polymerase chain reaction (PCR) and Single-strand conformation polymorphism (SSCP) PCR was performed by the method of Saiki et al.[9] as described previously[8].

Oligonucleotide primers used to amplify exons of factor VIII were as described in reference 10. The SSCP analysis was performed as described[11] and its gel-running conditions followed the procedures described by[6,7] with minor modifications[11] .

DNA sequencing. Asymmetric PCR amplification was performed by adding the two primers at a ratio of 1:20 or 1:50 to obtain single-stranded DNA fragments for direct sequencing[8]. The single-stranded DNA were purified and sequenced as described previously[8] using a third oligonucleotide primer complimentary to the single-stranded DNA[10].

RESULTS

Factor VIII gene is composed of 26 exons. Most of them are small and less than 300 bp except exon 14 which is around 3 kb. A total of 45 sets of oligonucleotides were synthesized to examine almost the entire coding region of factor VIII. We have used a recently developed technique called SSCP as a screening procedure to first identify the mutated exons and then determine the mutation by DNA sequencing. The SSCP stands for the single strand conformation polymorphism which allows the detection of DNA fragments of same size but different in just a single nucleotide. PCR derived factor VIII exons were labeled at their 5'-end with ^{32}P, denatured by formamide and analyzed by native acrylamide gel electrophoresis. The mutated DNA was identified by their distinct mobilities as a result of different conformation contributed by mutation in DNA sequence. Of 17 patients we have studied, 4 are mild to moderate and the remaining 13 are severe hemophilia A. Point mutations were identified for the 4 mild-moderate cases, resulting in missense mutations. Of the 13 severe hemophiliacs, 7 patients also revealed point mutations causing missense (3 cases) or nonsense mutations. The 3 missense variants occurred at residues 1689 (Arg-Cys, thrombin cleavage site), 1760 (Gly-Glu), and 1885 (Glu-Lys); and the 4 nonsense at residues 1796 (Gln) 1827 (Lys; 2 independent cases) and 1966 (Arg). The remaining 6 severe patients contained small deletions (3 cases), duplications (2 independent cases with identical duplications) and gross deletions (1 case, deleting exons 4-10 as judged by failure of PCR amplification of the lost exons).

It is conceivable that mutations which affect the factor VIII protein synthesis, such as gene (or nucleotide) deletions, duplications and nonsense mutations which create a stop codon and cause premature termination of translation, these will cause severe episode. The four missense mutations in that amino acid substitutions occurred and resulted in mild or moderate hemophilia, we found that the mutated residues are not conserved in factor VIII, factor V or ceruloplasmin, three homologous plasma proteins, or only conserved between factor VIII or factor V. While the amino acid substitutions resulting in severe hemophilia, are found at residues which are well conserved among factor VIII, factor V and ceruloplasmin.

Our study has allowed us to perform carrier detection by demonstration of the mutated exon by SSCP or the presence of the altered nucleotide sequence in the defective allele. Supported by grant no. NSC82-0412-B002-154M2, National Science Council, Taiwan.

REFERENCES

1. Haldane J.B.S. (1935) The rate of spontaneous mutation of a human gene. J. Genet. 31, 317-326.

2. Gitschier, J., Wood, W.I., Goralka, T.M., Wion, K.L., Chen, E.Y., Eaton, D.H., Vehar, G.A., Capon, D.J., and Lawn, R.M. (1984). Characterization of the human factor VIII gene. Nature 312: 326-330.

3. Toole, J.J., Knopf, J.L., Wozney, J.M., Sultzman, L.A., Buecker, J.L., Pittman, D.D., Kaukman, R.J., Brown, E., Shoemaker, C., Orr, E.C., Amphlett, G.W., Foster, W.B., Coe, M.L., Knutson, G.J., Fass, D.N., and Hewick, R.M. (1984). Molecular cloning of a cDNA encoding human antihaemophilic factor. Nature 312: 342-347.

4. Vehar, G.A., Keyt, B., Eaton, D.H., Rodriguez, H., O'Brien, D.P., Rotblat, F., Oppermann, H., Keck, R., Wood, W.I., Harkins, R.N., Tuddenham, E.G.D., Lawn, R.M., and Capon, D.J. (1984). Structure of human factor VIII. Nature 312: 337-342.

5. Wood, W.I., Capon, D.J., Simonsen, C.C., Eaton, D.H., Gitschier, J., Keyt, B., Seeburg, P.H., Smith, D.H., Hollingshead, P., Wion, K.L., Delwart, E., Tuddenham, E.G.D., Vehar, G.A., and Lawn, R.M. (1984). Expression of active human factor VIII from recombinant DNA clones. Nature 312: 330-337.

6. Orita, M., Iwahana, H., Kanazawa, H., Hayashi, K., and Sekiya, T. (1989a) Detection of polymorphisms of human DNA by gel electrophoresis as single-strand conformation polymorphisms. Proc. Natl. Acad. Sci. USA 86: 2766-2770.

7. Orita, M., Suzuki Y., Sekiya, T., and Hayashi, K. (1989b). Rapid and sensitive detection of point mutations and DNA polymorphisms using the polymerase chain reaction. Genomics 5: 874-879.

8. Lin, S.W., and Shen, M.C. (1991). Characterization of genetic defects of hemophilia B of Chinese origin. Thrombos Haemostas 66: 459-463.

9. Saiki, R.K., Scharf, S., Faloona, F., Mullis, K.B., Hort, G.T., Erlich, H.A., and Arnheim, N. (1985). Enzymatic amplification of β-globin genomic sequenced restriction site analysis for diagnosis of sickle cell anemia. Science 230: 1350-1354.

10. Lin, S.W., Lin, S.R., and Shen, M.C. (1993) Characterization of Genetic defects hemophilia A of Chinese origin. (Submitted)

11. Lin, S.W., and Shen, M.C. (1993). Genetic basis and carrier detection of hemophilia B of Chinese origin. Thromb and Haemost (in press).

POSSIBLE INVOLVEMENT OF PLATELET ACTIVATING FACTOR (PAF) IN TISSUE FACTOR GENERATION AND THE PATHOGENESIS OF DISSEMINATED INTRAVASCULAR COAGULATION (DIC)

Z. Terashita, M. Kawamura, Y. Imura, and K. Nishikawa

Research on Research, Pharmaceutical Research Division (ZT) and Department II of Pharmaceutical Research Laboratories I (MK, YI and KN), Takeda Chemical Industries, Ltd., 17-85, Juso-Honmachi 2-chome, Yodogawa-ku, Osaka, 532, Japan

INTRODUCTION

PAF is a highly potent lipid mediator with diverse biological actions such as activation of platelets and leukocytes, induction of hypotension and bronchoconstriction (1). In earlier papers, we reported that PAF may play important roles in the pathogenesis of anaphylactic shock in mice and endotoxin shock and DIC in rats using the first PAF antagonist, CV-3988 (2-5).

DIC is a pathological syndrome resulting from uncontrolled simultaneous activation of the blood coagulation and fibrinolytic systems. Diseases associated with DIC are sepsis, malignant tumors, obstetrical complications and others. In sepsis, DIC is commonly noted with Gram-negative infection due to endotoxin release. Endotoxin has diverse biological actions such as activation of platelets, leukocytes and the coagulation-fibrinolytic system and induction of synthesis of cytokines such as inter-leukin-1 (IL-1) and tumor necrosis factor (TNF), and chemical mediators including PAF (6). Tissue factor (TF) is a procoagulant glycoprotein that activates the extrinsic blood coagulation pathway in the presence of factor VIIa. Though a triggering role of TF in DIC has been suggested (6,7), the mediator(s) responsible for the induction of TF synthesis is not yet known.

In 1986, we presented our hypothesis that PAF may be involved in DIC caused by endotoxin (5). Recently, we succeeded in obtaining a novel PAF antagonist, TCV-309 {(3-bromo-5-[N-phenyl-N-2-[[2-(1,2,3,4-tetrahydro-2-isoquinolylcarbonyloxy)ethyl]carbamoyl]ethyl]carbamoyl]-1-propylpyridinium nitrate)} . The PAF antagonistic action of TCV-309 is over 100 times more potent than CV-3988 (8). Most recently, clinical investigations of TCV-309 have begun (9). In this paper, we further investigate the involvement of PAF in endotoxin-induced DIC in rats using TCV-309 (10).

MATERIALS AND METHODS

Endotoxin-induced DIC in rats: Experiments were done according to the methods described in our previous reports (5,10). In brief, male Sprague-Dawley rats, 6 to 9 weeks old, were anesthetized with sodium pentobarbital (50 mg/kg, i.p.), and endotoxin (0.25 mg/kg/hour) was infused at a rate of 0.6 ml/hour for 4 hours. TCV-309 (0.1 or 1 mg/kg) was given as follows: at first, 20% of the TCV-309 was given as a bolus (1 ml/rat) 5 minutes before the endotoxin infusion, and then the remaining

80% was coinfused with the endotoxin at rate of 0.6 ml/hr over 4 hours. In the normal group 0.9% saline was infused.

PAF-induced DIC symptoms in rats: PAF (15 μ g/kg/hour) was infused for 4 hours. TCV-309 (1 mg/kg) was given as described above.

Determination of DIC parameters: At the end of the infusion, 1.8 ml of blood was collected from the abdominal aorta using a citrate anticoagulant (final citrate concentration, 0.315%).This sample was used for the measurement of platelet count, activated partial thromboplastin time (APTT), prothrombin time (PT) and plasma fibrinogen level. An additional 1 ml of blood was taken without any anticoagulants for the measurement of fibrin and fibrinogen degradation products (FDP). These DIC parameters were measured as described in previous reports (5,10).

Determination of plasma TF activity: TF activity was measured according to the method of Fukuda et al. (11). In brief, the euglobulin fraction prepared from citrated plasma was dissolved in 30 mM barbital buffer (pH 7.35, containing 120 mM NaCl), heated for 3 minutes at 60 ℃ to denature factor Xa and fibrinogen and then centrifuged at 4 ℃. The supernatant (0.075 ml) was incubated with 0.15 ml of 50 mM Tris buffer (pH 7.5, containing 100 mM NaCl and 15 mM CaCl$_2$) for 5 min at 37 ℃ and then with PPSB solution (containing factor VII and factor X) for 10 minutes at 37 ℃. The reaction was stopped by the addition of 1.8 ml of ice cold 50 mM Tris buffer (pH 7.5, containing 100 mM NaCl and 2.5 mM EDTA). The activity of factor Xa was determined by the amidolytic activity using a chromogenic substrate, S-2222 (final concentration; 0.066 mM). TF activity was expressed by Xa activity.

Statistical analysis: Data was expressed as the mean±SEM. Williams Wilcoxon's test was used for the statistical analysis. A P value of less than 0.05 was considered significant.

RESULTS

Effects of TCV-309 on experimental DIC: The infusion of endotoxin caused DIC symptoms in rats (Fig. 1). The platelet count was significantly decreased, and PT and APTT were significantly prolonged. Plasma fibrinogen was decreased, whereas FDP was increased. The high dose of TCV-309 (1 mg/kg) partially but significantly improved all these DIC parameters. The low dose of TCV-309 (0.1 mg/kg) tended to improve them. The high dose of TCV-309 in itself had no effect on DIC parameters in normal rats.

Plasma TF activity in DIC rats and the effects of TCV-309: The endotoxin infusion caused a 25-fold increase in plasma TF activity from the normal value of 59±20 to 1453±187 nkat/l (Fig. 2). The high dose of TCV-309 inhibited the increase in plasma TF activity induced by endotoxin by 47%.

Effects of PAF infusion on DIC parameters: The infusion of PAF caused modest but significant changes in some DIC parameters: PT was increased from the normal value of 11.7±0.2 to 13.7±0.5 seconds, FDP was increased from <2.5 to 5.6±2.5 μ g/ml and fibrinogen was decreased from 3.1±0.3 to 2.2±0.2 mg/ml. Moreover, PAF caused a slight but significant increase in the plasma TF activity from the normal values of 27 ± 27 to 113 ± 27 nkat/l. TCV-309 (1 mg/kg) inhibited the PAF-induced changes in FDP, fibrinogen and TF activity and tended to inhibit the prolongation of PT (10).

<u>Histopathological examination</u>: In the kidney from DIC rats, massive fibrin deposition was observed in the glomerular capillaries. The high dose of TCV-309 clearly inhibited the glomerular fibrin deposition in the DIC rats (10).

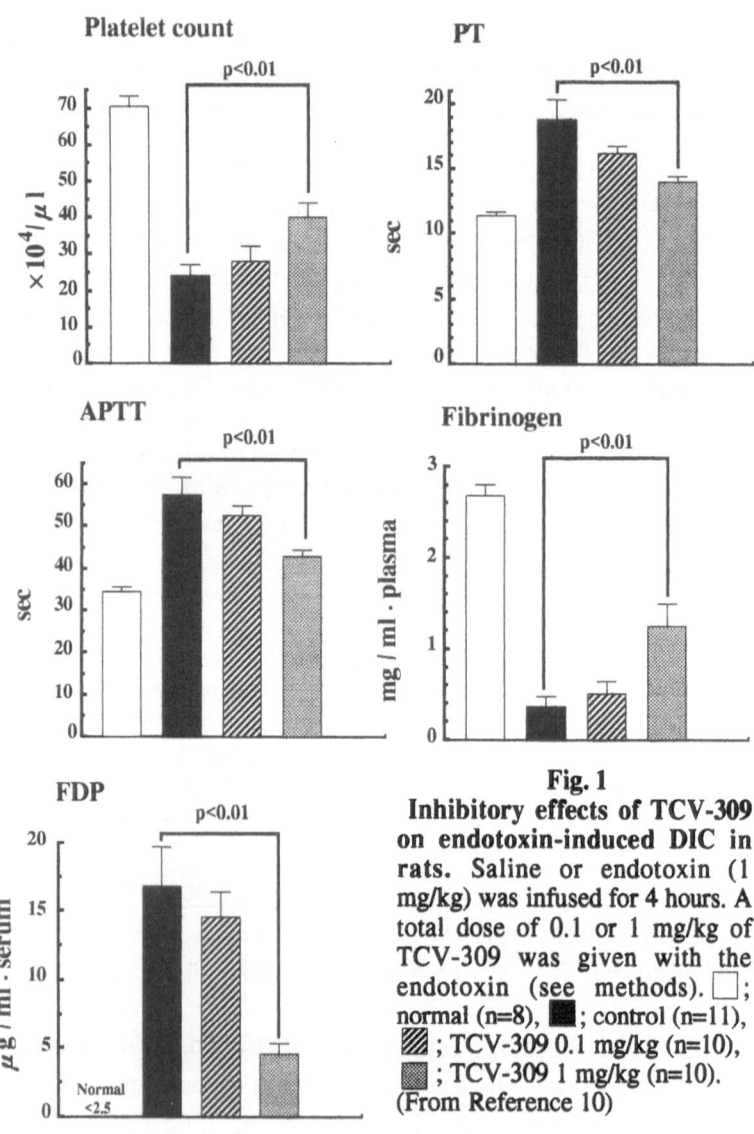

Fig. 1
Inhibitory effects of TCV-309 on endotoxin-induced DIC in rats. Saline or endotoxin (1 mg/kg) was infused for 4 hours. A total dose of 0.1 or 1 mg/kg of TCV-309 was given with the endotoxin (see methods). □; normal (n=8), ■; control (n=11), ▨ ; TCV-309 0.1 mg/kg (n=10), ▨ ; TCV-309 1 mg/kg (n=10). (From Reference 10)

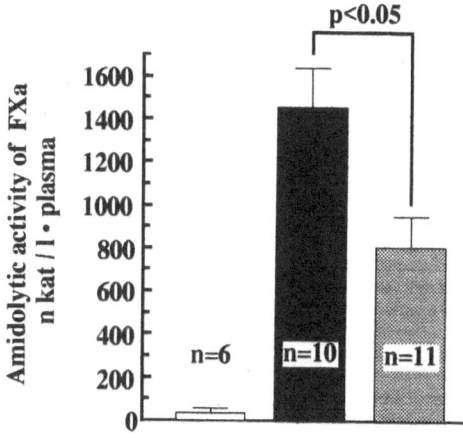

Fig. 2
Effect of TCV-309 on the change in plasma tissue factor activity in endotoxin-induced DIC in rats. Saline or endotoxin (1 mg/kg) was infused for 4 hours. A total dose of 1 mg/kg of TCV-309 was given with the endotoxin (see methods). □;normal, ■;control, ▨;TCV-309 1 mg/kg. (From Reference 10)

DISCUSSION

TCV-309 (1 mg/kg) significantly ameliorated the endotoxin-induced DIC symptoms such as decreases in platelet count and fibrinogen level, prolongation of PT and APTT, an increase in FDP (Fig. 1) and glomerular fibrin deposition (10) in rats. Therefore, we have confirmed the efficacy of PAF antagonists in the endotoxin-induced DIC in rats using TCV-309.

Though rat platelets lack the PAF-receptor (12), TCV-309 as well as CV-3988 significantly attenuated thrombocytopenia. There are at least two possible explanations for this phenomenon. First, PAF might prime the endotoxin-induced platelet activation or contribute to the generation of TNF during DIC. Priming effects of PAF on endotoxin-induced thrombocytopenia or lung injury via the production of TNF in rats have been reported (13,14). Second, platelets might be incorporated into thrombi during blood coagulation.

TCV-309 is a specific PAF antagonist: TCV-309 specifically and potently inhibits PAF-induced platelet aggregation, does not inhibit arachidonic acid metabolism and shows no antagonistic effects on vasoactive substances including bradykinin, leukotriene C_4, prostacyclin or thromboxane A_2 (8). TCV-309, therefore, ameliorate the DIC symptoms through its PAF antagonistic actions. To clarify the mechanisms of the beneficial action of PAF antagonists in DIC, we focused on the plasma TF activity in rats with DIC. Fukuda et al. established a method for the measurement of TF activity using S-2222 and demonstrated a marked increase in plasma TF activity in patients with DIC (11). We applied their method to rat plasma and found a great increase in plasma TF activity in DIC rats, and this increase was inhibited by TCV-309 (1 mg/kg) (Fig. 2). PAF also caused a slight but significant increase in plasma TF activity and changes in some DIC parameters. These changes were also inhibited by TCV-309.

TF is widely distributed in many tissues (1,2), however, it is not present in resting

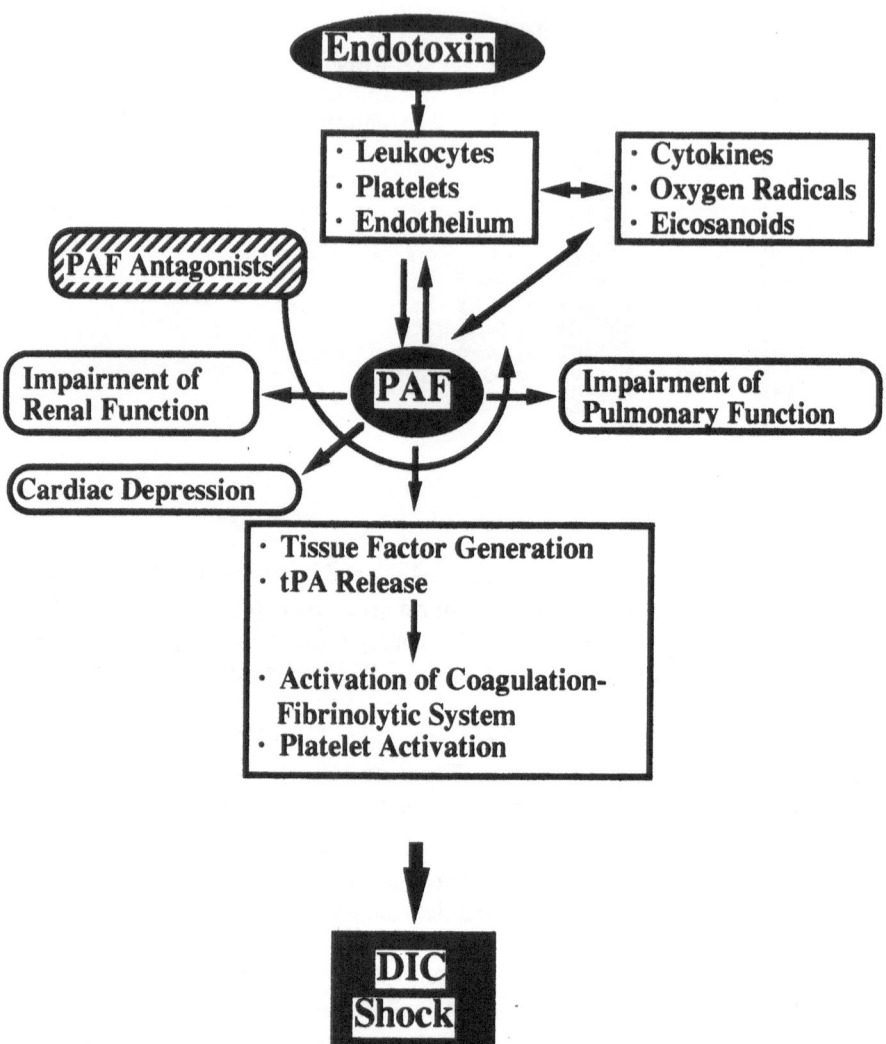

Fig.3 Possible involvement of PAF in the pathogenesis of DIC and shock

monocytes or endothelium. Various stimuli such as endotoxin and cytokines including IL-1 and TNF can induce the expression of TF in these cells (15,16). Therefore, the origin of plasma TF might be monocytes and endothelial cells. PAF and lipid A cause TF generation in macrophages, which is inhibited by a PAF antagonist (17). Furthermore, endotoxin stimulates biosynthesis of PAF in monocytes (18), and PAF potentiates the endotoxin-induced generation of IL-1 and TNF (13-16,19). Moreover, PAF causes the release of tissue-type plasminogen activator (tPA) (20). Thus, PAF can activate the blood coagulation-fibrinolytic system via the generation of TF and the release of tPA and can be involved in the pathogenesis of DIC. We did not measure the

PAF level in plasma or tissues. However, the plasma level of PAF, measured by gas chromatography-mass spectrometry, is greatly increased in patients with DIC (21).

Finally, we summarize the possible roles of PAF in the pathogenesis of DIC and shock caused by endotoxin based on the above findings and numerous studies using PAF antagonists (Fig. 3) (1,12). PAF antagonists may be useful drugs for the treatment of DIC and shock with sepsis.

References

1. Braquet, P., Touqoui, L., Shen, T.Y. and Vargaftig, B.B. (1987)   Pharmacol. Rev. 39: 97-145
2. Terashita, Z., Tsushima, S., Yoshioka, Y., Nomura, H., Inada. Y. and Nishikawa, K. (1983) Life Sci. 32: 1975-1982
3. Terashita, Z., Imura, Y., Nishikawa, K. and Sumida, S. (1985) Eur. J. Pharmacol. 109: 257-261
4. Terashita, Z., Imura, Y., Shino., A. and Nishikawa, K. (1987) J. Pharmacol. Exp. Ther. 243: 378-383
5. Imura, Y., Terashita, Z. and Nishikawa, K. (1986) Life Sci. 39: 111-117
6. Mullar-Berghaus, G. (1989) Semin. Thromb. Haemost. 15:58-86
7. Carson S.D. (1984) Prog. Clin. Pathol. 9:1-14
8. Terashita, Z., Kawamura, M., Takatani, M., Tushima, S., Imura, Y. and Nishikawa, K. (1992) J. Pharmacol. Exp. Ther. 260: 748-755
9. Stockmans, F., Arnout, J., Depre, M., Schepper, P.D., Angehrn, J.C. and Vermylen, J. (1991) Thromb. Haemost. 65: 1108P (Abst)
10. Kawamura, M., Terashita, Z., Imura, Y., Shino, A. and Nishikawa, K. (1992) Thromb. Res. in press.
11. Fukuda, C, Iijima, K and Nakamura K (1989) Clin. Chem. 35:1897-1990
12. Terashita, Z., Imura, Y. and Nishikawa, K. (1990) In: Handley, D.A., Saunders, R.N., Houlihan, W.J. and Tomesch, J.C. (Eds.) Platelet-activating factor in endotoxin and immune diseases. Marcel Dekker,Inc.New York. NY. pp 547-575
13. Pleszczynski, M.R. (1990) J. Lipd. Med. 2: S77-S82
14. Rabinovici, R., Esser, K.M., Lysko, P.G., Yue, T., Grisworld, D.E. Hillegass, L.M., Bugelski, P.J., Hallenbeck, J.M. and Feurstein,G(1991) Circ.Res.69:12-25
15. Gilmore, M.A. Proc. Natl. Acad. Sci. U.S.A. (1986) 83: 4533-4537
16. Tanaka, M. (1989) Thromb. Res. 56:201-211
17. Hirata, M., Shimomura, Y. and Yoshida, M. (1991) Thromb. Haemost. 65: 1107P (Abst)
18. Leaver, H.A., Qu, J.M., Smith, G., Howie, A., Ross, W.B. and Tap, P.L. (1990) Immunopharmacol. 20:105-113
19. Barett, M.L., Lewis, G.P., Ward, S., Westwick, J. (1987) Br. J. Pharmacol 90: 113P
20. Emeis, J.J. and Kluft, C. (1985) Blood 66: 86-91
21. Sakaguchi, K., Masugi, F., Chen, Y.H., Inoue, M., Ogihara, T. Yamada, K. and Yamastu, I. (1989) J. Lipid Med. 1: 171-173

PREVENTION OF VITAMIN K DEFICIENCY IN THE EARLY NEONATAL PERIOD

- PROPHYLACTIC ORAL ADMINISTRATION OF VITAMIN K (MK-4) TO PREGNANT CASES -

H. SHIMADA[1], E. TAKASHIMA[1], M. IKEUCHI[1], Y. ONO[1], T. HOSHINO[1], M. NONOGAKI[1],

M. YAMASHITA[1], K. PAKU[1], K. OHKURA[2], M. SOHMA[3] AND S. KASAKURA[3]

Department of Obsterics and Gynecology[1], Pediatrics[2] and Clinical Laboratory[3], Kobe City General Hospital, Kobe, Japan.

INTRODUCTION

To prevent vitamin K (VK) deficiency-related hemorrhage in infancy, the Committie on Nutrition of the American Academy of Pediatrics has recommended the prophylactic administration of VK to all newborns since 1961 [1], and so intramuscular injection of VK immediately after birth has been widely accepted in the USA but has not been uniformly practiced throughout the world for fear of neuromuscular complications. Intravenous injection of VK may also cause shock probably due to its solvent (CHO 60) [2]. Now in Japan, an oral administration of VK2 syrup (Kaytwo®, Eisai, Co., Ltd.) to newborns has been carried out since 1984. As a result, these ten years, the incidence of late hemorrhagic disease which occurs in infants after the first week from birth has decreased from 18/100000 deliveries to 2/100000 deliveries [3]. But the classic hemorrhagic disease of the newborn, occuring between 1 and 7 days old, namely melena neonatorum which is rather mild, and whose incidence is one hundred times more than that of the late hemorrhagic disease [1, 4]. This disease is still seen because the immediate administration of VK after birth to newborns has not yet widely accepted because of the risk of necrotizing enterocolitis [5] due to the high osmolarity of the syrup [6]. To prevent melena neonatorum, we have given mothers before delivery VK2 capsule orally (Kaytwo® capsule, Eisai. Co., Ltd.) containing 5mg of VK2, menaquinone-4 (MK-4), which was first put on the market in Japan in 1988. The present study was undertaken to evaluate the effect of prophylactic oral VK2-administration to the mothers according to the incidence of melena neonatorum and to redefine an effectively prophylactic dosage and administration time of VK2.

MATERIALS AND METHODS

We conducted this study from January, 1988 to April, 1992, and assigned 3606 pregnant cases of more than 37-week gestation to three groups : a non-medicated group (Group 1) and two medicated groups, one of which were orally administered with vitamin K2 in a dosage of 10mg /day (Group 2) and the other in a dosage of 20mg/day (Group 3) from 37-week gestation to delivery. If the mothers want to continue taking the drugs after delivery, the MK4-administration was permitted. Blood samples were collected from 182 mother-infant pairs at the time of delivery (Group 1, 83 cases, Group 2, 67 cases, Group 3, 32 cases) and protected from exposing light. The blood was mixed with 3.13% sodium citrate and centrifuged at 3000 g for 10 minutes and stored at $-20°C$ until it was used. Breast milk was collected from the cases in the three groups (Group 1, 80 cases , Group 2, 68 cases, Group 3, 34 cases) on the 3rd day of puerperium. Further, from 28 cases in Group 3 (15 cases with VK2 medication after delivery, and 13 cases without it after delivery), the breast milk was collected on the 3rd and the 5th day of puerperium. Concentrations of MK-4 in the plasma and breast milk were measured by the method using high performance liquid chromatography [7]. To evaluate the effect of the MK-4 administration to the mothers on the basis of the values from the Hepaplastin test (HPT) : Normotest (Owren) [8], We collected blood from the 5-day-aged neonates whose mothers belonged to Group 1 (59 cases) and Group 2 (77 cases).

RESULTS

MK-4 concentrations in the maternal and umbilical cord plasma

The mean MK-4 concentrations in the maternal plasma from the cases in Group 1, Group 2 and Group 3 were 0.24 ± 0.26 ng/ml, 1.64 ± 2.01 ng/ml and 3.88 ± 6.60 ng/ml, respectively. These concentrations of MK-4 in the maternal plasma were less than 0.1 ng/ml in 33 of 83 cases without the MK-4 administration (39.8%), while those of MK-4 were less than this value in only 2 of 99 cases with MK-4 the administration (2.0%) (Fig. 1. a).
The mean MK-4 concentrations in the umbilical cord plasma were 0.02 ± 0.06 ng/ml (Group 1), 0.16 ± 0.14 ng/ml (Group 2), 0.18 ± 0.23 ng/ml (Group 3), respectively. The concentrations of MK

-4 in the umbilical cord plasma were more than 0.1 ng/ml in 11 of 83 cases without the MK -4 administration (13.3 %), while those of MK-4 were more than this value in 69 of 99 cases with the MK-4 administration (69.7 %)   (Fig. 1. b.).

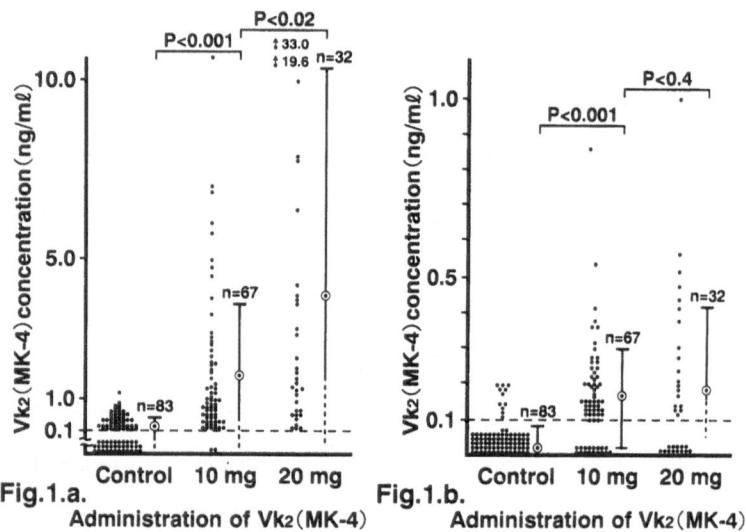

Fig.1.a.   Administration of Vk2(MK-4)

Fig.1.b.   Administration of Vk2(MK-4)

Fig.1. a. : Comparison of MK-4 concentrations in the maternal plasma at delivery between the groups with and without the MK-4 medication.
Fig.1. b. : Comparison of MK-4 concentrations in the umbilical cord plasma at delivery between the groups with and without the MK-4 medication.
Vertical bars and points show Mean ± SD. (Student's t test)

MK-4 concentrations in the breast milk on the 3rd day of puerperium

The mean concentrations in the breast milk from the cases in Group 1, Group 2 and Group 3 were 2.20 ± 4.31 ng/ml, 17.7 ± 20.6 ng/ml and 49.6 ± 57.9 ng/ml, respectively (Fig. 2. a).

MK-4 concentrations in the breast milk on the 3rd and the 5th day of puerperium

In the group with the MK-4 administration after delivery, MK-4 concentrations in the breast milk increased from the 3rd day to the 5th day after delivery, but in the group without MK-4 medication after delivery those decreased. There was a significant difference in the MK-4 concentrations in the breast milk on the 5th day of puerperium between groups with and without the medication after delivery ($p < 0.001$) (Fig. 2. b).

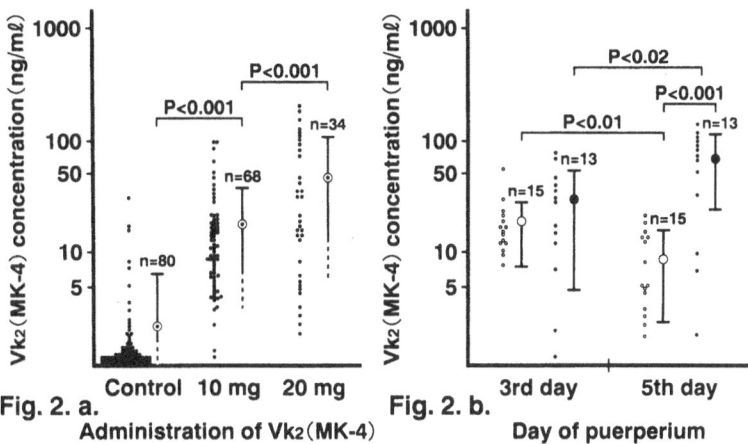

Fig. 2. a.
Administration of Vk₂(MK-4)

Fig. 2. b.
Day of puerperium

Fig. 2. a : Comparison of MK-4 concentrations in the breast milk on 5th day after delivery
between the groups with and without the MK-4 medication.

Fig. 2. b : MK-4 concentrations in the breast milk at the 3rd and the 5th day of puerperium
with and without the MK-4 medication after delivery. Open circles indicate the values
of the non-medicated group after delivery and closed circles indicate the values of
the medicated group after delivery. Vertical bars and points show Mean ± SD.
(Student's t test)

Comparison of the neonatal HPT values between the groups with and without the MK-4 medication

(10mg)

The mean values of HPT in the plasma of 5-day-aged newborns whose mothers were

administered with MK-4 and were not administered with MK-4 were $41.3 \pm 10.9\%$ and $37.3 \pm$

12.6%, respectively ($p < 0.05$). The incidence of the HPT values of less than 20% is 0% (0/77)

in the MK-4 treated group but 7% (4/59) in the MK-4 non-treated group ($p < 0.05$) (Table. 1).

Table. 1. The values of HPT in the plasma of 5 day-aged newborns with and without
administration of MK-4 (10mg).

Administration of VK₂ (10mg)	No of cases	Values of HPT (M ± SD)	Incidence of HPT of less than 20%
No	59	37.3±12.6% ⎤ P<0.05	4 (7%) ⎤ P<0.05
Yes	77	41.3±10.9% ⎦	0 (0%) ⎦

Values : Student's t test
Incidence : x^2 test

<u>Incidence of melena neonatorum</u>

In this study, we had tested 3606 cases of more than 37-week gestation out of 3891 cases of total deliveries. While there was only one case of melena neonatorum in the groups administered with 10mg/day or 20mg/day of MK-4 orally from 37-week gestation (1/1526, 0.07%), this disease were seen in 15 cases in the control group without antenatal MK-4 medication (15/2080, 0.72%). Melena neonatorum occured in only one baby whose mother had been treated with MK-4 for one day and a half (Table. 2).

Administration of VK$_2$		No of Deliveries	No of Melena neonatorum	
Non		2080	15 (0.72%)	
dosage	10mg	1305	1	P<0.01
	20mg	221	0	
	total	1526	1 (0.07%)	

Table 2. Prophylactic administration of VK2 and the incidence of melena neonatorum. (x^2 test)

DISCUSSION

Based on the measurements of various forms of VK in the amniotic fluid, meconium, maternal and umbilical cord plasma, Hiraike has reported that VK1 and VK2, especially MK-4, may have important physiological functions for the fetus [9]. MK-4 is more effective than VK1 on the hemostasis [10]. Therefore, we gave VK to the mother as the form of MK-4. We reported that MK-4 was transported to the baby through the placenta effectively and safely [11]. In this report, we also showed clinically that a significant decreace of the incidence of melena neonatorum was due to the medication of MK-4 to the mother before delivery. These findings are supported by the improved laboratory data from the neonates, i.e., the fact the incidence of the HPT values of less than 20% is 0% in MK-4 treated group even if the dosage of MK-4 is 10mg/day. We are not able to expect to record the date of delivery precisely, and so we started VK medicaiton from 37-week gestation. It is unknown how many hours or days it takes for MK-4 given orally to the mothers to act in the fetus. But our investigation shows that we have to give Kaytwo® capsules to the mother for at least 2 days before delivery because only one case of melena neonatorum seen in MK-4 treated group was medicated with MK-4 for one and a half day. It is also shown that the concentration of MK-4 accumulated in the breast milk decrease rapidly when MK-4 administration is stopped after delivery. If we expect the effect of MK-4 on the prevention of late hemorrhagic disease, it may be necessary to continue the medication after delivery. This study suggests that prenatal oral administration of MK-4 to the mother is useful in preventing melena neonatorum and that the medication of MK-4 after delivery takes the place of the oral administration of Kaytwo® syrup to the baby at the time of discharge because of the transportation of MK-4 through the breast milk.

REFERENCES

1. Committee on Nutrition, American Academy of Pediatrics. (1961) Pediatrics 28 : 501-507.

2. Hama R, Morihisa Y. (1986) The Informed Preacriber (in Jpn) 1 : 9-12.

3. Hanawa Y. (1992) Acta Paediatr Jpn 34 : 107-116.

4. Maki M. (1991) Haemostasis and Thrombosis in Obstetrics and Gynecology.
    Die Medizinische Verlagsgesellschaft mbH, Germany. pp 202-217.

5. Torma MJ, Delemos LA, Rogers CR, Diserens HW. (1973) Am J Surg 126 : 758-761

6. Ukita A, Takahashi A, Nunotani T, Nishizawa K, Takakura K, Emi N, Kibana T,
    Tanaka M, Nakata E, Kameyama J. (1986) J Obst Gynec Neonat Hematol (in Jpn)
    10 : 455-463.

7. Yamano Y, Ikenoya S, Tsuda T, Ohmae M, Kawabe K. (1977) YAKUGAKU ZASSHI
    97 : 486-494.

8. Owren PA, Strandli OK. (1969) Særtrykk av farmakoterapi 25 : 14-26.

9. Hiraike H, Kimura M, Itokawa Y. (1988) Am J Obstet Gynecol 158 : 564-569.

10. Tajima T, Ohgoh T, Miyao K. (1971) Folia Pharmacol japon 67 : 478-485.

11. Shimada H, Himeno K, Michimoto T, Tanada S, Ikeuchi M, Suwa M, Ono Y, Hoshino T,
    Takashima E, Ohkura K, Sohma M, Maeda Y, Kasakura S. (1990) Acta Obst Gynaec Jpn
    42 : 705-710.

THE EFFECT OF ARGATROBAN ON THE ABILITY OF GLYCEROL TO INHIBIT CEREBRAL
EDEMA AND THE EFFECT OF THE CO-ADMINISTRATION OF ARGATROBAN WITH T-PA AND
HEPARIN ON BLLEDING TIME

K. TANABE, Y. HONDA AND M. IWAMOTO
Exploratory Research Laboratories II, Daiichi Pharmaceutical Co., Ltd.,
Tokyo 134, Japan.

INTRODUCTION

Glycerol, which is a low molecular weight (92 g/mol) alcohol, may
enter the brain at a very slow rate; therefore, its administration will
raise blood osmolality and create an osmotic gradient between plasma and
brain with resultant net removal of water from brain. Indeed, previous
studies showed that it appears to be an effective cerebral dehydrating
agent [1-5].
Argatroban, which has specific affinity for thrombin [6,7], inhibits
fibrin formation and thrombin-stimulated platelet aggregation [8-11].
Argatroban is clinically effective for inhibition of occurrence and
progression of thrombosis, such as cerebral thrombosis [12] or peripheral
arterial occlusive disorders. As the therapy for cerebral thrombosis,
glycerol is often used to inhibit cerebral edema induced by the thrombosis. Therefore, it is important to examine whether or not the drug
interferes with the ability of glycerol. In this study, we used a rat
cerebral thromboembolism model and investigated the effect of argatroban
on the ability of glycerol.
On the other hand, tissue-type plasminogen activator (t-PA) has been
shown to specifically activate plasminogen in the presence of fibrin [13]
and to be a more potent thrombolytic agent than urokinase in vitro [14].
As the therapy for acute myocardial infarction by t-PA, heparin is used
in order to inhibit the blood coagulation which would possibly occur by
cathether insertion into coronary artery for infusion of t-PA. Recently,
argatroban becomes to be administered together with t-PA and heparin in
the therapy for myocardial infarction to prevent reocclusion. In this
case, hemorrhage might be a severe side-effect because thrombolytic agent
and anticoagulant drugs are co-administered. If the combined treatment
does not cause a severe hemorrhage, argatroban would be useful in the
therapy for myocardial infarction. In the present study, we also investigated the effect of the combined treatment on bleeding time in rabbits.

MATERIALS AND METHODS

Materials   Glyceol (fructose-added glycerol solution: 10% glycerol, 5%
fructose, 0.9% sodium chloride) was purchased from Chugai Pharmaceutical
Co., Ltd. Japan. Bovine serum albumin (fraction V) was purchased from
Daiichi Pure Chemicals, Japan. Argatroban was the product of Mitsubishi
Chemical Industries, Ltd. Japan. Argatroban was mixed with saline or
glyceol at a concentration of 0.1 mg/ml and incubated for 10-15 min in
the water at 56°C to dissolve.
The TD-2061 (recombinant human tissue-type plasminogen activator,
5,000,000 IU/1 vial) employed was the product of Toyobo Co., Ltd. Japan
and was dissolved in saline. Heparin (1,000 U/ml) was mixed with saline
at a concentration of 100 U/ml.

Animals   Male Wistar rats weighing 230-280 g and male New Zealand White
rabbits weighing 2.1-3.3 kg were used.

Part I. The effect of argatroban on the ability of glycerol to inhibit
cerebral edema
(1)Preparation of blood clot fragments   Blood clot fragments were prepared following a slight modification of the method described by Hara et
al. [15].   Rats were anesthetized with sodium thiopental (100 mg/kg,
i.p.).   Five ml of blood was obtained from the carotid artery and kept at
room temperature to clot.   The blood clot and serum were transferred into
a syringe and the clot was fragmented by passing it several times through
needles, first a 25 gauge needle, second a 26 gauge, and finally a 27
gauge.   The blood clot fragments were washed on a metal net (mesh size
200) four times with 25 ml of isotonic saline containing 1% of bovine
serum albumin.   Then, the fragments were resuspended in rat serum to
obtain suspension with blood clot fragment protein concentration of 7.5
mg/ml, as measured by the Lowry method [16] in the serum.

(2)Procedures for embolization   Embolization in a cerebral vessel was
induced according to the method of Hara et al. [15].   Rats were anesthetized with halothane, and the internal and external right carotid arteries were exposed.   The external artery was occluded with a thread and the
common carotid artery was temporarily occluded with a clip about 15 mm
below the bifurcation.   A 100 ul sample of the blood clot fragment suspension containing 7.5 mg/ml protein was injected into the common carotid
artery using a 26 gauge needle.   After injection, the needle was withdrawn and the site of injection was sealed off with surgical adhesive
(Alon-Alfa, Sankyo, Japan).   The clip on the common carotid artery was
removed and the flow was restored.   Argatroban and/or Glyceol was infused
over 2 hr into the femoral vein immediately after the injection of clot
under halothane anesthesia (10 ml/kg/hr or 20 ml/kg/hr).   After the
infusion, the animals were killed by decapitation under halothane anesthesia and the brain was removed.   The rats which received not the infusion but the clot injection were made to come out from under the anesthesia immediately after clot injection and then were killed by decapitation
at 2 hr after clot injection.

(3)Brain water measurement   To obtain measurement of brain water, the
content of each cerebral hemisphere was measured using the differences
between the wet and dry weights of the tissue [17].   Each cerebral hemisphere was weighed and then dried at 120°C for 18-24 hr.   The amount of
evaporated water was calculated and the result was expressed as the
percentage of water in the tissue.
   water content (%)
   = ((wet weight - dry weight)/wet weight) x 100

(4)Analysis of data   The statistical significance of data was analysed by
the Tukey (b) test.   A p value of <0.05 was considered significant.   Data
are presented as means $\pm$ S.E.

Part II. The effect of the co-administration of argatroban with t-PA and
heparin on bleeding time
(1)Animal model   Rabbits were anesthetized with sodium thiopental.   At
first 0.3-0.5 ml of sodium thiopental solution (100 mg/ml in saline)
was injected into the marginal ear vein carefully, and then 2 ml of the
solution was injected i.p..   Additional anesthetic was administered as
needed.
   In case of t-PA administration, a catheter was placed in the femoral
vein for continuous infusion of t-PA.   Then, t-PA infusion (2 ml/kg/hr)
began 60 min prior to the measurement of bleeding time.   The infusion was
continued till when the measurement of bleeding time was over.
   In case of co-administration of t-PA with argatroban and heparin, two
catheters were placed in both femoral veins for continuous infusion of
t-PA and argatroban.   Then, t-PA infusion (2 ml/kg/hr) began 60 min prior
to the measurement of bleeding time. Argatroban infusion (0.4 mg/2
ml/kg/hr) began 30 min prior to the measurement of bleeding time.   At 5
min prior to the measurement of bleeding time, heparin (100 U/ml/kg)

was bolus injected into the marginal ear vein. The infusion was continued till when the measurement of bleeding time was over.

(2)Measurement of bleeding time Standard cuts were made in the ear artery of one ear at the length of 1 cm using a 22 gauge needle attached to a syringe containing 0.1 ml of sodium citrate solution (3.1%), and 0.9 ml of blood was aspirated without force. Then, the needle was drawn out and the measurement of the bleeding time was begun. A filter paper was blotted with the blood every 15 seconds. The bleeding time was the interval from when the needle was drawn out to when the blood did not seep through the paper.

(3)Hematological tests Activated partial thromboplastin time (APTT) and prothrombin time (PT) were measured by the use of thromboplastin reagent (Organon Teknika Corporation).

(4)Analysis of data The statistical significance of data was analysed by the Kruskal-Wallis test. If the signficant difference was found, the data was analysed by the Wilcoxon test. A p value of <0.05 was considered significant. Data are presented as means $\pm$ S.E.

RESULTS

Effects of glyceol and/or argatroban on contralateral cerebral water content Contralateral or ipsilateral cerebral water contents when glyceol and/or argatroban were administered are shown in Table 1. Infusion of glyceol reduced significantly the water content (C vs. E; p<0.01) although the increase of contralateral cerebral water content by the injection of clot was not observed (A vs. B; p>0.05). Argatroban treatment (2.0 mg/kg/2 hr) showed no effect on the ability of glyceol to reduce cerebral water content (E vs. F; p>0.05). And argatroban itself did not affect cerebral water content (C vs. D; p>0.05).

Table 1. Effects of glyceol and/or argatroban on water content of brain tissue

		n	Contra.[h] (percentage water)	Ipsi.[i] (percentage water)
A[a]	Untreated control	9	79.36$\pm$0.14	79.23$\pm$0.11
B[b]	Clot only	9	79.59$\pm$0.30	80.26$\pm$0.24
C[c]	Clot + saline	10	79.52$\pm$0.17	80.17$\pm$0.17
D[d]	+ argatroban	5	79.34$\pm$0.30	79.80$\pm$0.35
E[e]	+ glyceol	9	78.22$\pm$0.08	78.99$\pm$0.10
F[f]	+ argatroban + glyceol	4	78.83$\pm$0.26	78.89$\pm$0.18
G[g]	+ 1/2 glyceol	5	79.09$\pm$0.23	80.04$\pm$0.45

a; Untreated control
b; Clot injection control
c; Clot injection + saline infusion (20 ml/kg/2 hr)
d; Clot injection + argatroban (in saline) infusion (2 mg/20 ml/kg/2 hr)
e; Clot injection + glyceol infusion (20 ml/kg/2 hr)
f; Clot injection + argatroban (in glyceol) infusion (2 mg/20 ml/kg/2 hr)
g; Clot injection + glyceol infusion (10 ml/kg/2 hr)
h; Contralateral hemisphere
i; Ipsilateral hemisphere
Data represents mean $\pm$ S.E..
Significant differences between groups were observed as below.
  Contra.; A vs. E (p<0.01), B vs. E (p<0.01), C vs. E (p<0.01),
          D vs. E (p<0.01)
  Ipsi. ; A vs. B (p<0.05), A vs. C (p<0.05), B vs. E (p<0.01),

B vs. F (p<0.05), C vs. E (p<0.01), C vs. F(p<0.05),
E vs. G(p<0.05)

Effects of glyceol and/or argatroban on ipsilateral cerebral water content   Ipsilateral cerebral water content at 2 hr after the injection of clot increased significantly (A vs. B; p<0.05), and infusion of glyceol (20 ml/kg/2 hr) suppressed significantly this increase (C vs. E; p<0.01). Argatroban treatment (2.0 mg/kg/2 hr) showed no effect on the ability of glyceol to reduce cerebral water content (E vs. F; p>0.05). And argatroban itself did not affect cerebral water content (C vs. D; p>0.05).

Effects of t-PA on bleeding time   Table 2 shows the effects of t-PA on bleeding time, APTT or PT.   When t-PA   (100,000, 300,000, 1,000,000 IU/kg/hr) was infused for 1 hr in rabbits,   the prolongation of bleeding time, APTT or PT was not observed.

Table 2. Effects of t-PA on bleeding time

	n	BT[a] (sec)(%)	APTT (sec)	PT (sec)
t-PA				
Control	11	162+15(100)	145.4+8.1	7.3+0.4
20,000 IU/kg/hr	7	144+14(88)	-	-
100,000 IU/kg/hr	7	148+12(91)	-	-
300,000 IU/kg/hr	5	129+12(79)	153.3+11	7.2+0.3
1,000,000 IU/kg/hr	5	159+24(98)	142.0+10	7.1+0.2

[a]; Bleeding time
Data represents mean + S.E..
Significant differences between groups were not observed.

Table 3. Effects of co-administration of t-PA with heparin and argatroban on bleeding time (t-PA; 100,000 IU/kg/hr)

	n	BT[a] (sec)(%)	APTT (sec)	PT (sec)
t-PA	5	120+25(100)	100.4+14	8.4+0.5
t-PA + heparin	5	147+18(123)	>452.3##	12.7+1#
t-PA + argatroban	4	165+19(138)	151.2+36	11.5+1#
t-PA + heparin + argatroban	5	198+43(165)	>500##	16.8+2##

[a]; Bleeding time
Data represents mean + S.E.. # p<0.05 vs. t-PA
p<0.01 vs. t-PA

Effects of co-administration of t-PA with heparin and/or argatoban   on bleeding time (1)   Table 3 shows the effects of co-administration of t-PA (100,000 IU/kg/hr) with heparin and/or argatroban on bleeding time, APTT or PT.   When t-PA   was co-administered with   heparin (100 U/kg), the prolongation of bleeding time, APTT or PT was observed than when t-PA only was administered.   Similarly, when t-PA   was co-administered with argatroban (0.4 mg/2 ml/kg/hr), the prolongation of bleeding time, APTT or PT was   observed.   And when   t-PA   was co-administered with heparin (100 U/kg) and argatroban (0.4 mg/2 ml/kg/hr), the additive prolongation of bleeding time was observed.   This prolongation was not significant.

Effects of co-administration of t-PA with heparin and/or argatroban   on bleeding time (2)   Table 4 shows the effects of co-administration of t-PA (1,000,000 IU/kg/hr) with heparin   and/or argatroban   on bleeding time, APTT or PT.   When t-PA was co-administered with   heparin (100 U/kg), the shortening of the bleeding time was observed though the pro-

longation of APTT or   PT was observed.   When t-PA   was co-administered
with argatroban (0.4 mg/2 ml/kg/hr), the prolongation of bleeding time
was not observed though the prolongation of APTT or   PT was observed.
Similarly, when   t-PA   was co-administered with heparin (100 U/kg) and
argatroban (0.4 mg/2 ml/kg/hr), the prolongation of bleeding time was not
observed though the prolongation of APTT or PT was observed.

Table 4. Effects of co-administration of t-PA with heparin and argatroban
on bleeding time (t-PA; 1,000,000 IU/kg/hr)

	n	BT^a (sec)(%)	APTT (sec)	PT (sec)
t-PA	5	210+35(100)	143.6+2.5	10.7+0.4
t-PA + heparin	4	150+8.7(71)	>500#	14.1+0.7#
t-PA + argatroban	5	189+7.6(90)	183.5+5.4#	12.6+0.6#
t-PA + heparin + argatroban	5	186+32(89)	>500##	17.8+2##

^{a}; Bleeding time
Data represents mean + S.E..   # p<0.05 vs. t-PA
                          ## p<0.01 vs. t-PA

DISCUSSION

In this study, we used a rat cerebral thromboembolism model in which
blood clot fragments were introduced into the carotid artery.   In this
model, the clot was injected into the internal right carotid artery.
Therefore, ipsilateral cerebral water content   increased more than contralateral cerebral water content by the injection.   Ipsilateral cerebral
water content at 2 hr after the injection of clot increased significantly, and infusion of glyceol (20 ml/kg/2 hr) suppressed significantly this
increase.   Infusion of glyceol reduced significantly the water content
although the increase of contralateral cerebral water content by the
injection of clot was not observed.   These results suggest that glycerol
reduced water content of both normal brain and wet brain.
Argatroban treatment (2.0 mg/kg/2 hr) showed no effect on the ability
of glyceol to reduce cerebral water content.   And argatroban itself did
not affect cerebral water content. These results indicate that argatroban
could be administered together with glycerol for the patients with cerebral thrombosis.
In clinic, t-PA is administered at a dose of 20,000 IU/kg/hr or
1,000,000 IU/kg/hr for acute cerebral thrombosis or acute myocardial
infarction, respectively.   The prolongation of bleeding time was not
observed at these doses in rabbits and therefore it is suggested that t-
PA at the dose used in clinic has no effect on hemorrhage.
When 100,000 IU/kg/hr of t-PA was co-administered with heparin or
argatroban, the prolongation of bleeding time was observed than when t-PA
only was administered.   And when t-PA was co-administered with heparin
and argatroban, the additive prolongation of bleeding time was observed.
On the other hand, when 1,000,000 IU/kg/hr of t-PA was co-administered
with heparin and/or argatroban, the prolongation of bleeding time was
not observed. The reason of this phenomenon is unclear, but polysorbate
80 which is contained in the solution of t-PA might be concerened.
In this study, we found that co-administration of t-PA with heparin and
argatroban did not prolong the bleeding time more than that of t-PA with
heparin in rabbits.   Co-administration of argatroban with other drugs
could be used widely in clinical application.

KEYWORDS

argatroban, glycerol. t-PA, heparin, bleeding time

REFERENCES
1. Absolon MJ (1966) Brit J Ophthalmol 59: 683-688
2. Buckell M, Walsh L (1964) Lancet 2: 1151-1152
3. Cantore GP, Guidetti B, Virno M (1965) J Neurosurg 21: 278-283
4. Mathew NT, Meyer JS, Rivera VM, Charney JZ, Hartmann A (1972)
   Lancet 2: 1327-1329
5. Newkirk TA, Tourtellotte WW, Reinglass JL (1962) Arch Neurol
   27: 95-96
6. Okamoto S, Hijikata A, Kikumoto R, Tonomura S, Hara H,
   Ninomiya K, Maruyama A, Sugano M, Tamao Y (1981)
   Biochem Biophys Res Commun 101: 440-446
7. Kikumoto R, Tamao Y, Tezuka T, Tonomura S, Hara H, Ninomiya K,
   Hijikata A, Okamoto S (1984) Biochemistry 23: 85-90
8. Tamao Y, Yamato T, Hirata T, Kinugasa M, Kikumoto R (1986)
   Jpn Pharmacol Ther suppl 14: 869-874
9. Hara H, Tamao Y, Kikumoto K (1986) Jpn Pharmacol Ther suppl
   14: 875-881
10. Green D, Ts'ao C-H, Reynolds N, Kahn H, Cohen I (1985)
    Thromb Res 37: 145-153
11. Esumi N, Todo S, Imashyuku S (1987) Cancer Res 47: 2129-2135
12. Kobayashi S, Kitani M, Yamaguchi S, Suzuki T, Okada K,
    Tsunematsu, T (1989) Thromb Res 53: 305-317
13. Hoylaerts M, Rijken DC, Lijken HR, Collen D (1982) J Biol Chem
    257: 2912-2919
14. Matsuo O, Rijken DC, Collen D (1981) Thromb Haemost 45: 225-229
15. Hara T, Iwamoto M, Ogawa H, Yamamoto A, Tomikawa M (1990)
    Thromb Res 59: 703-712
16. Lowry OH, Rosebrough NJ, Farr AL, Randall, RJ (1951) J Biol Chem
    193: 265-275
17. Shigeno T, Brock M, Shigeno S, et al. (1982) J Neurosurg
    57: 99-107.

EFFECTS OF ANTICOAGULANTS ON THROMBOLYSIS MEDIATED BY TISSUE PLASMINOGEN ACTIVATOR IN EXPERIMENTAL THROMBOSIS MODEL

Katsumi Nakagawa, Hajime Tsuji, Keizo Yamada, Mitsuru Yoneda, Osamu Takada, Yuka Yamada, Haruchika Masuda, Masashi Uno, Toshiyuki Tamagaki, Masahito Yamagami, Kazuharu Katoh, Katsumi Yamamoto, Kyoichiro Kobayashi, Shohei Sawada and Masao Nakagawa

Second Department of Medicine, Kyoto Prefectural University of Medicine, 465 Kajii-cho Hirokoji Kawaramachi, Kamigyo-ku, Kyoto 602, Japan

INTRODUCTION

Tissue plasminogen activator (t-PA) is being used as thrombolytic therapy for patients with acute myocardial infarction [1], given in combination with anticoagulants such as heparin or warfarin. We compared the effects of the new selective thrombin inhibitors, argatroban and hirudin, with those of heparin, on the thrombolysis mediated by t-PA in an experimental model of thrombosis using the hamster cheek pouch.

MATERIALS AND METHODS

Male golden Syrian hamsters weighing 120 to 130g were anesthetized with pentobarbital sodium (100 mg/kg ip). After tracheotomy, the right subclavian artery and right femoral vein were both cannulated to allow drug administration. The microvasculature of the right cheek pouch was prepared for direct microscopic and photographic observation using the method of Shanberge et al [2]. Five minutes after the injection of fluorescent sodium (50 mg/kg) through the right subclavian artery, a selected venule measuring 50 to 70 μm in diameter was irradiated by filtered light (20 mW/mm^2, wave length; 400-500 nm) until the developing thrombus stenosed 99% of the luminal area.

Thirty minutes after the thrombus formation, we administered t-PA (TD-2061; TOYOBO, 72x10^4 IU/kg·hr) continuously through the right subclavian artery, either alone or in combination with unfractionated heparin (UFH; Kabi, 12.5 U/kg·hr), recombinant hirudin (Hir; Sigma, 1500 U/kg·hr) or with argatroban (Arg; MD-805, Mitsubishi Chemical Ind. Ltd., 0.05, 0.1, 0.2 and 0.3 mg/kg·hr) through the right femoral vein. Control animals received an infusion of saline.

The microscopic image of the thrombus was photographed with a high gain video color camera (Flovel Co.Ltd.) and monitored and recorded on video.

The recorded configuration of the thrombus was transferred to the computed image analyzer (XL-500; AVIONICS) to evaluate the thrombolytic effects of each medication. The percent stenosis of the vascular lumen by the thrombus (%SL) was calculated as $\%SL = (H_{1\text{-}4}/D_0) \times 100$. The percent area of the thrombus (%AT) was calculated as $\%AT = (A_{1\text{-}4}/A_0) \times 100$. In those calculations, D_0 is the internal diameter of the vessel, H is the height of the thrombus and A is the area of the thrombus (Fig.1).

Coagulation tests such as prothrombin time (PT) and activated partial thromboplastin time (aPTT) were performed on plasma samples obtained one hour after the injection of the test medications.

In statistical analysis, differences between each treatment group were analyzed by the Williams-Wilcoxon test. Data are expressed as mean ± standard error (SE). A level of $p<0.05$ was accepted as statistically significant.

Key Words: tissue plasminogen activator (t-PA), argatroban, hirudin, heparin, thrombolysis

RESULTS

Thrombus Formation

After the injection of fluorescent sodium through the right subclavian artery, thrombus was produced with high reproducibility at the site that was irradiated with filtered light (Fig.1).

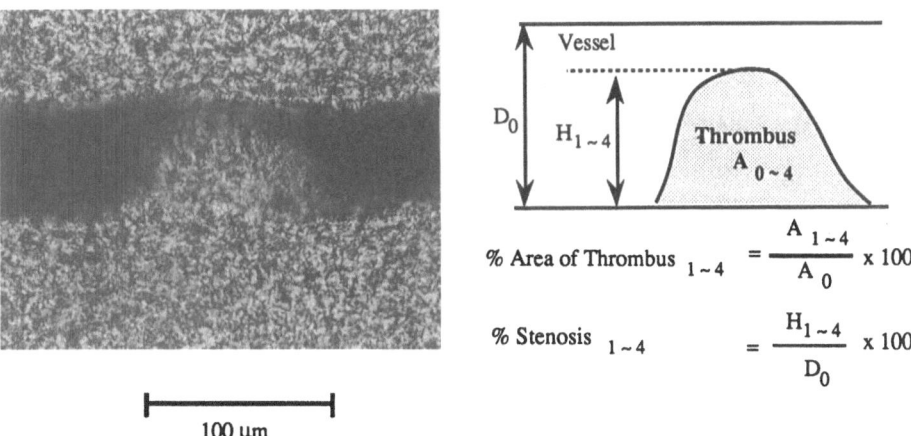

$$\% \text{ Area of Thrombus }_{1\sim4} = \frac{A_{1\sim4}}{A_0} \times 100$$

$$\% \text{ Stenosis }_{1\sim4} = \frac{H_{1\sim4}}{D_0} \times 100$$

Fig. 1 <u>Photographic and Schematic Representation of Thrombus</u>
Following the injection of fluorescent sodium (50 mg/kg), the irradiation of a selected venule (70 μm) by filtered light (20 mW/mm^2) produced a thrombus, that blocked 99% of the luminal area (shown at left). The percent stenosis of the lumen by the thrombus (%SL) and the percent areas of the thrombus (%AT) were each calculated as shown on the right. D_0: internal diameter of vessel, H: height of thrombus, A: area of thrombus.

Thrombolytic Process

The percent stenosis of the vascular lumen produced by the thrombus (%SL) and the percent area of the thrombus (%AT) in the control group decreased to 71.5±1.0% and 71.3±1.8%, respectively, in 4 hours. The continuous administration of t-PA through the right subclavian artery significantly reduced thrombus size. However, during the administration of the plasminogen activator, formation of a new thrombus was observed on the surface of the existing thrombus. Its size transiently increased causing a transient reocclusion (data not shown). This finding is common in another experimental thrombosis model [3]. Therefore, to achieve a more constant thrombolysis, we studied the efficacy of the anticoagulant on thrombolysis.

Anticoagulant Equivalence

Before comparing the effects of UFH, hirudin and argatroban in vivo, we measured PT and aPTT to determine the concentration of each drug to obtain an equivalent anticoagulant activity. UFH 12.5 U/kg·hr, Hir 1500 U/kg·hr and Arg 0.3 mg/kg·hr had an equivalent effect on the prolongation of PT and aPTT (Fig.2). Thus those doses were used in the following study.

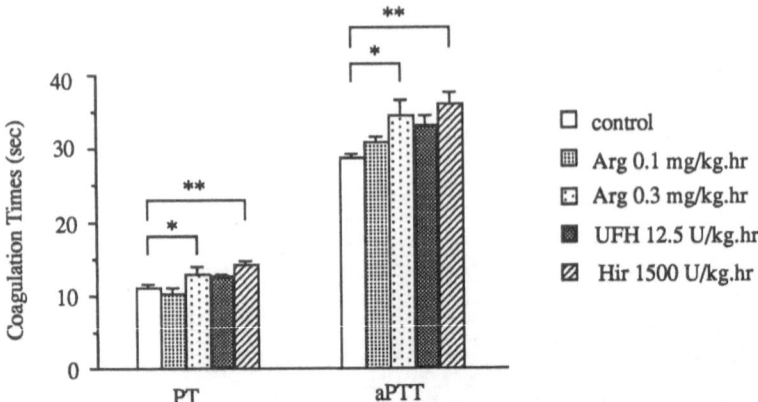

Fig. 2 Coagulation Times

Doses of unfractionated heparin 12.5 U/kg·hr, hirudin 1500 U/kg·hr and argatroban 0.3 mg/kg·hr produced an equivalent effect on PT and aPTT. PT: prothrombin time, aPTT: activated partial thromboplastin time, Arg: Argatroban, UFH: unfractionated heparin, Hir: Hirudin. Data represent mean±SE, n=5. **: $p<0.01$, *: $p<0.05$.

Additive Effect of Unfractionated Heparin on Thrombolysis Produced by t-PA

The effects of hirudin and argatroban were compared with those of UFH. Hirudin, similar to argatroban, effectively enhanced the thrombolytic effects of t-PA. In contrast, UFH decreased the effects of t-PA with significance (Fig.3). The combined administration of argatroban and t-PA in different doses was investigated. Argatroban dose dependently enhanced the thrombolytic effect with significance. One and two hours, the injection of argatroban 0.1, 0.2 and 0.3 mg/kg·hr, besides 0.05 mg/kg·hr, significantly decreased the percent of stenosis and the area of thrombus compared with the injection of t-PA alone (Fig.4).

DISCUSSION

Heparin is widely used to enhance the fibrinolytic efficacy of t-PA. However, reports indicate that it interferes with the fibrinolytic system in vitro [4]. Our findings agree with those obtained in other experimental models showing the inferiority of heparins over a selective thrombin inhibitor. UFH delayed the thrombolysis mediated by t-PA, whereas hirudin and argatroban significantly enhanced it. Argatroban is a selective and reversible inhibitor of thrombin [5]. Several mechanisms are associated in the difference in the efficacy between UFH and argatroban. First, they differ as to molecular size, and thus, in their accessibility to the interstices of the thrombus and to the thrombin exposed on its surface. Argatroban is much smaller than heparin, ATIII, or heparin-ATIII complex [6]. Second, heparin's inhibition of thrombin largely depends on ATIII: the higher level of thrombin which occurs during thrombosis and thrombolysis could lead to a depletion of ATIII. Under such circumstances, the administration of heparin would be less effective than giving a direct thrombin inhibitor [6]. Third, argatroban inhibits the generation of factor XIIIa and suppresses the extent of fibrin cross-linking, leading to an easier thrombolysis [7]; heparin lacks such a mechanism. Moreover, heparin has been reported to interfere with the fibrinolytic system at the surface of activated platelets by inhibiting the binding of t-PA and plasminogen to platelets [8].

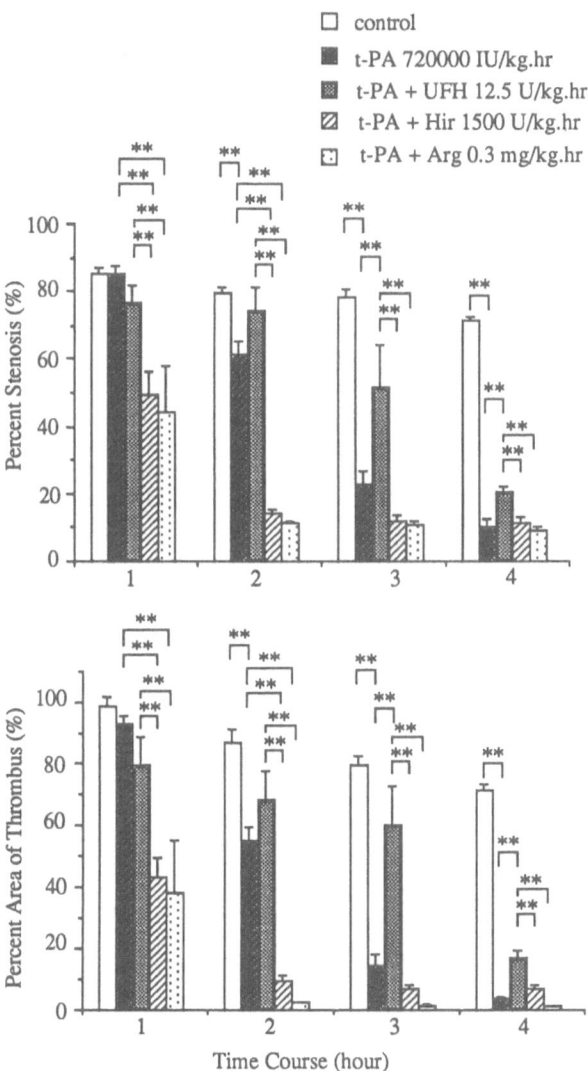

Fig. 3 <u>Additive Effects of Anticoagulants on Thrombolysis with t-PA</u>
Hirudin reacted similarly to argatroban and effectively enhanced t-PA thrombolysis. In contrast, UFH delayed t-PA thrombolysis as compared with t-PA alone, and vs Hirudin and Argatroban. t-PA: tissue plasminogen activator, Arg: Argatroban, UFH: unfractionated heparin, Hir.: Hirudin. Data represent mean±SE, n=4. **: p<0.01.

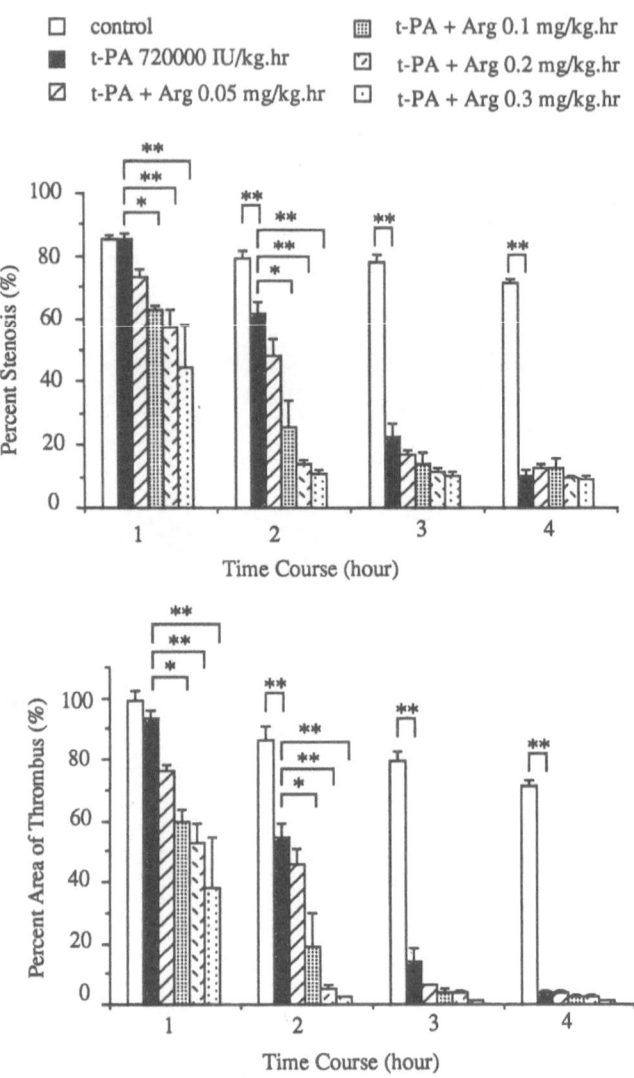

Fig. 4 Effects of Argatroban on Thrombolysis with t-PA
Administration of t-PA effectively enhanced the thrombolysis vs control. Argatroban enhanced the thrombolysis induced by t-PA, dose dependently and significantly in one and two hours after the injection. t-PA: tissue plasminogen activator, Arg: Argatroban. Data represent mean±SE, n=4. **: p<0.01, *: p<0.05.

Recombinant hirudin, a newly developed specific inhibitor of thrombin, is isolated from medicinal leeches [9]. It inhibits all the effects of thrombin resulting from its proteolytic activity, and is able to neutralize the thrombin exposed on the fibrin surface. Hirudin effectively inhibits the formation of fibrin on the surface of the dissolving thrombus, and thus enhances the thrombolytic effect of t-PA as shown in our findings.

CONCLUSION

Hirudin and argatroban effectively enhanced the thrombolysis mediated by t-PA, while conventional UFH delayed it. From these observations, it appears that a selective thrombin inhibitor may be a useful addition to thrombolytic therapy with plasminogen activator. Clinical studies are indicated in this respect.

REFERENCES

1. Marder VJ, Sherry S. (1988) Thrombolytic therapy: current status. N Engl Med 318: 1512-1520
2. Shanberge JN, Tsuji H, Longe TQ. (1990) Production of thrombi on intact endothelium by use of antiheparins in vivo. J Lab Clin Med 116: 831-839
3. Ik-Kyung Jang, Herman K. Gold, Robert C. Leinbach, John T. Fallon and Desire Collen. (1990) In vivo thrombin inhibition enhances and sustains arterial recanalization with recombinant tissue-type plasminogen activator. Circ Res 67: 1552-1561
4. Gaffney PJ, Marsh NA, Thomas DP. (1982) The influence of heparin and heparin-like substances on the fibrinolytic system in vivo. Heamostasis 12: 85
5. Okamoto S, Hijikata A. (1981) Potent inhibition of thrombin by the newly synthesized arginine derivative No.805. The importance of stereostructure of its hydrophobic carboxamide portion. Biochem Biophy Res Commun 101: 440-446
6. Rosenberg RD. Heparin-antithrombin system. In: Hemostasis and Thrombosis: Basic Principles and Clinical Practice. Colman RW, Hirsch J, Marder VJ, Salzman EW (eds). JP Lippincott, Philadelphia, PA 1987; pp 962-85
7. Tamao Y, Yamamoto T, Kikumoto R, Hara H, Itoh J, Hirata T, Mineo K, Okamoto S. (1986) Effect of a selective thrombin inhibitor MCI-9038 on fibrinolysis in vitro and in vivo. Thromb Heamostas 56: 29-34
8. Gorog P, Ridler CD, Kovacs IB. (1990) Heparin inhibits spontaneous thrombolysis and thrombolytic effect of both streptokinase and tissue-type plasminogen activator. An in vitro study of the dislodgement of platelet-rich thrombi formed from native blood. J Int Med 227: 125-132
9. Heras M, Chesebro JH, Penny WJ Bailey KR, Badimon L, Fuster V. (1989) Effects of thrombin inhibition on the development of acute platelet-thrombus deposition during angioplasty in pigs. Heparin versus recombinant hirudin, a specific thrombin inhibitor. Circulation 79: 657-665

The relationship between plasma fibronectin receptor levels and preeclampsia

Naohiro Kanayama and Toshihiko Terao
Department of Obstetrics and Gynecology, Hamamatsu University School of Medicine3600 Handa-cho, Hamamatsu, 431-31, Japan

key words, fibronectin receptor, pregnancy, abruptio placentae, integrin

INTRODUCTION

The cause of preeclampsia is still unknown, but is thought to be mainly endothelial injury. The endothelin, fibronectin levels of the maternal plasma increase in preeclampsia, indicating that endothelial cells are injured[1-2]. Fibronectin receptor (FNR) is an integrin that play important roles in cell-cell, interactions, cellular adhesion to an extracellular matrix and formation of a thrombus. FNR also appear on endothelial cells and it is closely related to their functions. Katayama et al. detected FNR in serum and found that its concentration was high in liver diseases[3]. However, there is no report on plasma FNR in pregnant women. In the present study we examine levels of plasma FNR during normal pregnancy, and in preclampsia and abruptio placenta.

MATERIALS AND METHODS

Plasma was obtained from 35 normal pregnant women diagnosed by routine check at different gestational ages; 1st trimester=0-13 weeks(n=5), 2nd=14-26 weeks(n=7), 3rd=27-delivery(n=23). Plasma were obtained by 19 gauge needle without using a tourniquet not to contaminate platelet-derived FNR and endothelial FNR. In addition 20 samples were obtained from patients with moderate(blood pressure 140-160/90-110 and 0.1-1.0g/day proteinuria) or severe preeclampsia (blood pressure more than 160/110, proteinuria more than 1g/day) in the 3rd trimester and 8 samples from patients at the onset or within 24 hours before the onset of abruptio placentae (in the 3rd trimester). Of these cases of abruptio placentae, 6 had moderate or severe preeclampsia, and 2 had no preeclampsia. Plasma was also obtained sequentially for 10 days until separation from 2 patients with abruptio placentae. We could observe these two patients continuously due to admission for preeclampsia. These three groups did not differ significantly in parity or age. The patients with preeclampsia were treated by bed rest and diet control(NaCl 6g/day, 1800 Cal/day) and those with severe preeclampsia were also given hydralazine. Details of samples from patients with abruptio placentae are shown in Table 1. Plasma were stored at -80 ° C until examined.

The concentration of FNR was measured with an enzyme-linked immunoabsorbent assay kit from Takara Shuzou (Tokyo, Japan). Briefly, 96-well plates were coated overnight at 4 ° C with monoclonal FNR antibody (FNR5), which recognized only the β_1 subunit of FNR receptor, in 0.2 M Na_2CO_3 buffer, pH 9.6. This antibody did not react with other β_1 subunit of integrins. The wells were then washed with phosphate buffered saline (PBS), and blocked with 2 % bovine serum albumin in PBS (90 min, 37° C). After washing again, 50 μ l of various concentrations of standard FNR purified from human placenta (purity 98%) or of plasma was added and the plates were incubated for 60 min at 23 ° C with peroxidase labeled monoclonal FNR antibody (FNR2), which also reacts with the β_1 subunit of FNR. The plates were then washed 5 times with PBS and incubated for 10 min at 37 °

C with 100 μl of o-phenylenediamine-HCl. The reaction was stopped by adding 1 N H$_2$SO$_4$, and the optical density at 492 nm was measured with a BIORAD EIA reader. All samples were examined in duplicate. Significance of differences were analysed by Student's t test. P value less than 0.05 provided significant difference.

D-Dimer was measured by Dimer test(Bering berke, Germany), thrombin antithrombin complex(TAT) and platelets counts were measured for preeclampsia.

The distribution of FNR in the placenta was examined immunohistochemically by the alkaline phosphatase-antialkaline phosphatase method. All placentas from cases of abruptio placentae, 4 placentas from cases of preeclampsia and 7 normal placentas obtained at delivery were examined. In this study we used FNR monoclonal antibody.

RESULTS

Results on the levels of FNR are shown in Fig 1. In normal pregnancy, the mean value of FNR was 1.4± 0.4μg/ml in the 1st trimester n=5 (0-13 weeks), 1.4 ±0.2 μg/ml in the 2nd n=7 (14-26 weeks), and 1.9±0.3 μg/ml(P<0.05) in the 3rd n=23 (27-delivery). Its level increased with pregnancy. During puerperium, the concentration decreased with time being 1.4± 0.5μg/ml on day 1, 1.0±0.3 μg/ml on day 2 and 0.8 ± 0.2μg/ml on day 3. In preeclampsia patients the level was 2.0 ±0.4 μg/ml, and in patients with abruptio placentae, it was 2.7 ±0.4 μg/ml(P<0.01 for normal pregnany and preeclampsia). The level in abruptio placentae was significantly higher than those in the other groups. The mean value of abruptio placentae with preeclampsia (2.9 ±0.3 μg/ml) was higher than that in abruptio placentae without preeclampsia (2.3μg/ml).

The correlation coefficients with FNR of preeclampsia were -0.35 for platelet 0.43 for d-dimer, and 0.32 for TAT (fig.2).

We followed 2 cases (cases 1 and 4) of abruptio placentae for 10 days until the onset of abruptio placentae, and the observed changes of FNR are shown in Fig 3A and Fig 3B. The FNR value was stable until 3 or 4 days before abruptio placentae, but inreased markedly before abruptio placentae occurred. In those patients, the change in FNR level differed from the changes of the platelet count (Fig.3A) and of other hematological parameters such as the level of D-dimer (Fig.3B), the prothrombin time and the partial thromboplastin time (not shown).

The results of immunohistochemical studies are summerized in table 2. Moderate staining for FNR was observed on the surface of decidual cells. Syncytial cells also stained for FNR(fig 4a). In preeclampsia, the surface of decidual cells stained strongly for FNR, and the chorionic villi stained weakly(fig. 4b). In abruptio placentae associated with preeclampsia, the surface and the area around decidual cells stained strongly, especially close to the hematoma(fig. 4c). In abruptio placentae without preeclampsia, decidual cells stained weakly(not shown).

DISCUSSION

De Strooper et al. reported the immunolocalization of the β_1 chain of the FNR in placental tissues and noted that FNR was localized to the apices of trophoblasts[4]. However, they did not describe FNR of decidua in detail and there are no reports of plasma FNR levels of pregnancy so far. We found that the plasma concentration of FNR increased during pregnancy from in the first trimester 1.4± 0.4μg/ml to in the third trimester 1.9±0.3 μg/ml. Adhesive proteins such as fibronectin, collagen and fibrinogen are known to be required for attachment and implantation of the placenta. Moreover, with increase in size of the placenta during gestation, larger amounts of these adhesive proteins and their receptors should be required. This would explain why the plasma FNR level increases with gestational age. Moreover, the plasma FNR concentration decreased immediately after delivery. These findings suggest that the increase in plasma FNR during pregnancy is mainly due to its production by the placenta.

The mean value of FNR in preeclampsia $(2.0 \mu g/ml)$ was higher than that of normal pregnant women in the third trimester. On histological examination, thrombi and fibrinoid degradation (decidua necrosis) are often observed in decidual tissue in preeclampsia[5]. We found that decidual and endothelial cells of cases of preeclampsia stained more strongly than those of normal pregnant women for FNR. Therefore, some pathological change of decidual tissue in preeclampsia may cause production of FNR on decidual cells and its release into the maternal circulation. In preeclampsia, FNR may be produced markedly in not only decidual endothelial cells but also endothelial cells in other vessels, because the main cause of preeclampsia is a endothelial damage of whole body. There were not significant correlation coefficients between FNR and other markers for preeclampsia. Platelet, d-dimer and TAT are thrombus related markers. As FNR may be released from endothelial cells or fibroblasts below the basement membrane, the change of FNR would be different from that of thrombus related markers. Anyhow FNR would be a sensitive and unique marker for preeclampsia.

We found that the plasma FNR concentration increased before abruptio placentae to much higher levels than those in normal pregnant women or preeclampsia cases. As on immunohistochemistry, decidua and placental villi stained for FNR strongly(data not shown), such tissues would be also sources of FNR. These findings suggest that the increased amount of plasma FNR in abruptio placentae is chiefly derived from the early separation site of the placenta, that is the wound of decidual tissue. Therefore, a marked increase of FNR in the maternal circulation seems to be one sign of early placental abruption.

We conclude from this study that the plasma FNR level is a new marker of preeclampsia and that marked increase of FNR is a sign of abruptio placentae.

REFERENCES
1. Mastrogiannis D.S., O'Brien W.F., Krammer J. and Benoit R. (1991) Potential role of endothelin-1 and hypertensive pregnancies. Am J Obstet Gynecol .159:908-914
2. Brubaker D.B., Ross M.G. and Marinoff D. (1992) The function of elevated plasma fibronectin in preeclampsia. Am J Obstet Gynecol. 166:526-531.

3. Katayama M., Kurome T., Yamamoto K., Uchida H., Hino F. and Kato I. (1991) Sandwich enzyme immunoassay for serum integrins using monoclonal antibodies. Clin Chim Acta. 202:179-190.

4. Strooper B.D., van der Schueren B., Jaspers M., Saison M., Spaepen M., van Leuven F., van den Berghe H. and Classimam J.J. (1989) Distribution of the β_1 subgroup of the integrins in human cells and tissues. J Histochem Cytochem. 37:299-307.

5. Kitzmiller J.L. and Benirscke K. (1973) Immunofluoresent study of placental bed vessels in preeclampsia of pregnancy. Am J Obstet Gynecol. 115:248-251.

Table 1. Characteristics of 8 cases of
abruptio placentae

Case	Age	Parity	Gesta-tional week	Pre-eclampsia	Plasma FNR μg/ml	Platelets before AP × 10⁴/mm³
1	22	0	29	severe	3.1	6
2	31	0	33	severe	2.9	18
3	26	2	37	severe	2.8	25
4	26	0	35	moderate	2.9	16
5	29	1	38	moderate	2.6	15
6	37	1	31	moderate	2.8	20
7	29	1	27	no preeclampsia	2.3	25
8	23	0	34	no preeclampsia	2.2	19

AP = Abruptio placentae.

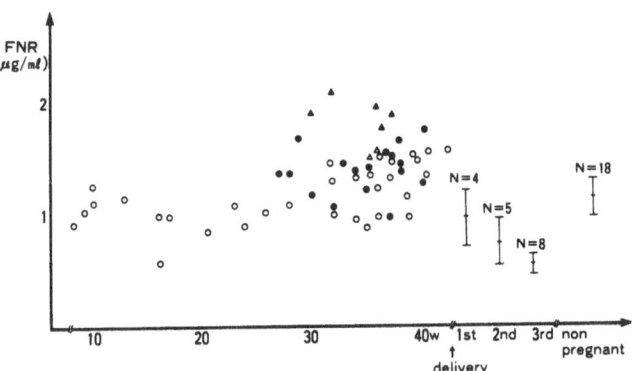

Fig. 1 FNR concentrations in women during pregnancy and the postpartum period. Open circles, normal pregnancy, closed circles, preeclampsia, open triangles, abruptio placentae without preeclampsia; close triangles, abruptio placentae with preeclampsia.

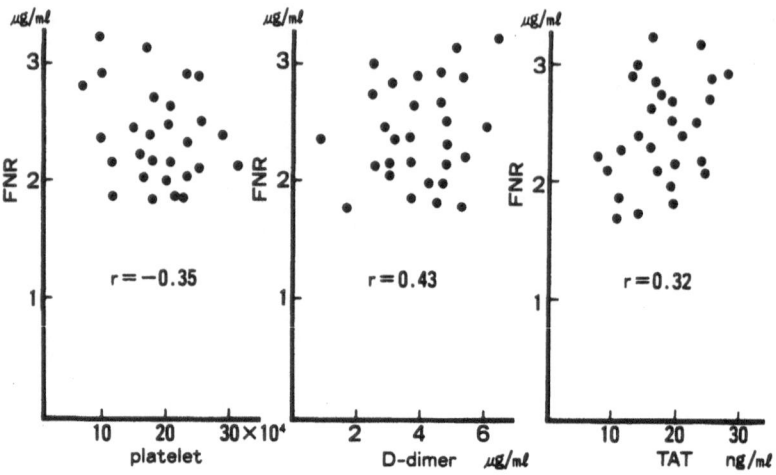

Fig. 2 The correlation coefficients between FNR and platelet, D-dimer, and thrombin-antithrombin complex (TAT).

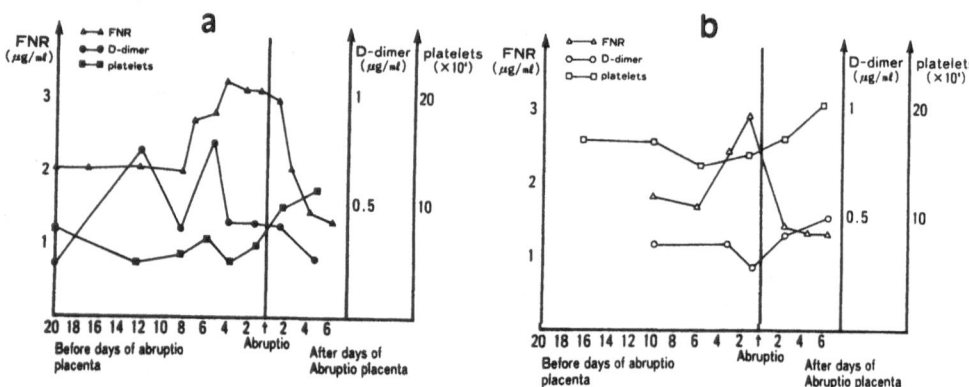

Fig. 3 Changes of FNR, D-dimer and platelet counts in abruptio placentae. 3A, case 1; 3B, case 4. Note that FNR increases before separation.

Fig.4 Photomicrograph of FNR localization. 4A, normal placenta at term. Decidual cell membranes and syncytial cells are stained moderately. 4B, placenta of a case of preeclampsia. Decidual cell membranes are strongly stained but syncytial cells are stained only weakly. 4C, placenta of a case of abruptio placentae. Decidual cells and their extracellular matrix are strongly stained, especially around the hematoma.

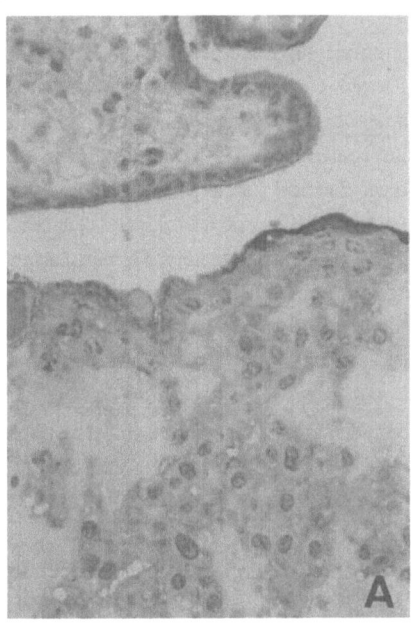

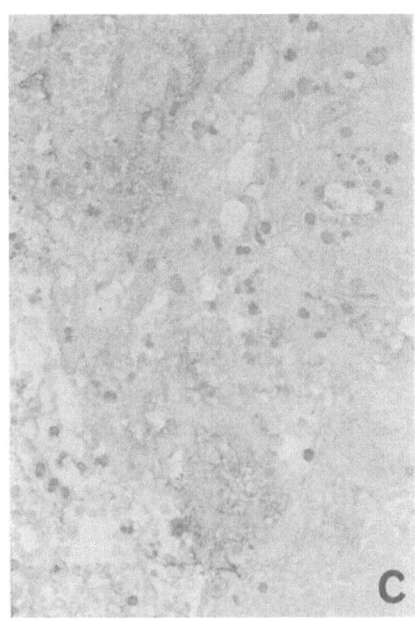

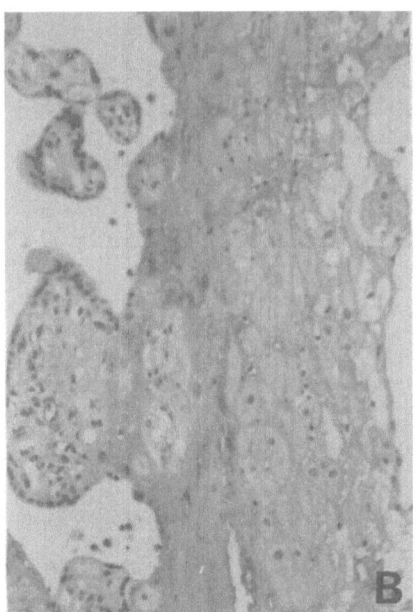

Table 2. FNR staining of decidua and syncytial cells

	Case	Gestational weeks	Cell membrane of decidual cells	Around decidual cells
Normal		14	++	–
(n = 7)		34	+	–
		37	+	–
		38	+	–
		38	++	–
		39	++	+
		40	++	–
Preeclampsia		31	+++	–
(n = 4)		33	+++	+
		37	++	+
		38	++	–
Abruptio	1	29	+++	+++
placentae	2	33	+++	+++
(n = 8)	3	37	+++	++
	4	35	+++	+++
	5	38	++	+++
	6	31	+++	+++
	7	27	++	+
	8	34	+	++

– = No staining; + = weak staining; ++ = moderate staining; +++ = intense staining.

Y. YOSHIZAWA, Y. SHINOZAKI, S. IZAKI AND K. KITAMURA

Department of Dermatology, Saitama Medical Center, Saitama Medical School, 1981 Kamoda, Tsujido, Kawagoe, Japan, 350.

INTRODUCTION

When the patients with herpes zoster (HZ) have severe underlying diseases or being treated with immunosuppressive agents, they may occasionally develop severe complications such as disseminated intravascular coagulation (DIC) or encephalitis [1,2]. Histopathological examination of herpetic lesion revealed that endothelial cells are damaged, suggesting that some mechanism takes place to induce hypercoagulable condition in this disease [2,3]. However, effects of varicella zoster virus (VZV) infection to coagulation and fibrinolysis system have not been fully documented. This study investigates changes of platelet count and hemostatic and fibrinolytic molecular markers. Influencing factors to hemostatic and fibrinolytic conditions such as location and size of lesions, dissemination, and pleocytosis of cerebrospinal fluid were analyzed. The age of the patient was found to be crucial factor to modify hemostatic and fibrinolytic changes in HZ.

Key Words: herpes zoster, platelet count, hemostatic and fibrinolytic molecular marker, cerebrospinal fluid pleocytosis

MATERIALS AND METHODS

Patients were admitted within 7 days after the onset of HZ and they received drip infusion of acyclovir for 5 to 7 days. Table 1 summarized the profile of patients.

Table 1. Patients examined in this study

	Number of patients	Mean age (range)	Distribution trigeminal	spinal	Patients with dissemination
Total	42	52 (5-79)	14	28	10
A*	23	50 (20-79)	10	13	8
B**	35	54 (20-79)	12	23	9

* Patients examined for molecular markers.
** Patients examined for CSF cell count.

Percent herpetic area The herpetic lesion on the spinal nerve region was traced on a paper for measurement of area and the ratio to total body surface was calculated.

Platelet count was estimated at acute phase and convalescence during the course of HZ respectively and the ratio of platelet decrease was expressed as follows.

$$(Plt_C - Plt_A) / Plt_C \times 100 \ (\%)$$

Plt$_C$: platelet count at convalescence

Plt$_A$: platelet count at acute phase

<u>Determination of hemostatic and fibrinolytic markers</u> Citrated blood was collected between 8 and 9 a.m. within 7 days after the onset. After centrifuging the plasma samples were quickly frozen and kept at -20° C until experiments. Plasma level of thrombin antithrombin III complex (TAT) was determined with ELISA technique according to the instructions of the manufacturer (TEIJIN, Japan). In the same way, α_2-plasmin inhibitor plasmin complex (PIC, TEIJIN, Japan), and fibrin degradation products D dimer (DD dimer, BMY, France) were assayed using the ELISA technique according to the instructions, as well.

<u>Cerebrospinal fluid (CSF)</u> was collected from the patients within 9 days after the onset. Diagnosis of pleocytosis was made when the cell count/field was over 30/3.

<u>Statistics</u> The differences in mean were assessed by analysis of variance (Anova) by means of application, Stat View II.

RESULTS

Platelet count in acute phase of HZ (Plt$_A$ 21.2±4.8/mm^3) was found decreased, when compared to the value in convalescence (Plt$_C$ 29.2±6.8/mm^3, p=0.0001). Although both degree of herpetic area and location of herpetic lesion did not affect the platelet decrease, a clear distinction was observed when the patients were separated between the cases with and without disseminated herpetic lesions: cases with dissemination showed greater decrease of platelet count (with dissemination vs without dissemination, 36.3±11.5% vs 25.1±12.5%, p<0.05, Table 2). The degree of platelet decrease was correlated with the level of TAT (r=0.63, p<0.05) or DD dimer (r=0.78, p<0.005, Fig. 1) in the patients without dissemination.

Table 2. Hemostatic and fibrinolytic molecular markers in herpes zoster

	Total	Trigeminal lesion	p*	Spinal lesion	with Dissemination	p**	without Dissemination
Platelet decrease (%)	28.5±13.7	32.8±14.9	(NS)	25.3±11.5	36.3±11.5	(<0.05)	25.1±12.5
TAT (ng/ml)	3.8±1.7	3.8±1.2	(NS)	3.9±2.0	4.6±1.9	(NS)	3.4±1.4
PIC (μg/ml)	0.8±0.5	0.7±0.4	(NS)	0.8±0.6	0.9±0.3	(NS)	0.7±0.6
DD dimer (ng/ml)	175±190	132±128	(NS)	211±230	204±196	(NS)	158±192

* Probability between patients with trigeminal lesion and those with spinal lesion
** Probability between patients with and without dissemination

It was noticed that there were a few persons who showed abnormally high level of molecular markers especially in aged female patients (67 years old female, TAT 8.6, DD dimer 673; 78 years old female, TAT 6.8, DD dimer 707; 77 years old female, TAT 4.6, DD dimer 454; 20 years old male, TAT 5.7, DD dimer 33). Therefore we plotted the degree of platelet decrease, level of TAT, PIC and DD dimer versus the age of the patients. When the platelet decrease was plotted versus the age of patients without dissemination a correlation to the age of patients was found. More significant platelet decrease was observed with the age when patients were over 40 years old (r=0.52, p<0.05) and more platelet decrease was observed when patients were younger than 40 years old (r= -0.79, p<0.01, Fig. 2).

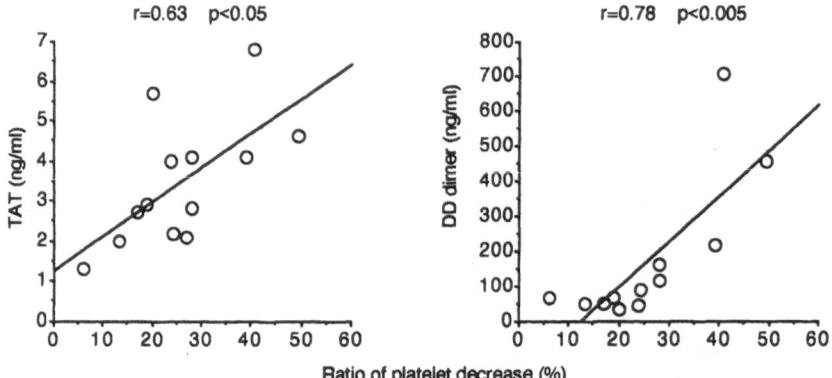

Fig. 1   Correlations of platelet decrease to level of TAT or DD dimer in the patients without dissemination

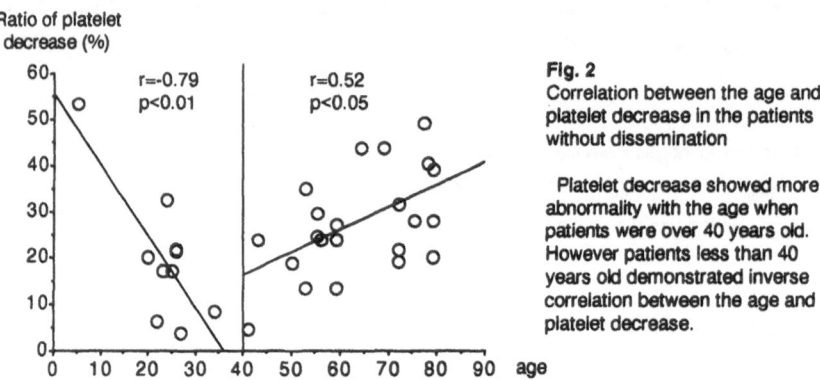

Fig. 2
Correlation between the age and platelet decrease in the patients without dissemination

Platelet decrease showed more abnormality with the age when patients were over 40 years old. However patients less than 40 years old demonstrated inverse correlation between the age and platelet decrease.

CSF samples showed pleocytosis in 49% of patients (Table 3). The mean of the cell count was 167/3 with the range of 0/3 and 992/3. The level of pleocytosis in the patients with dissemination was higher than those in the patients without dissemination (p<0.05). We, then, plotted the level of pleocytosis versus the age of patients without dissemination. A correlation was observed between the CSF cell count and the age (r=0.47, p<0.05, Fig. 3). Similarly, a correlation was observed between the platelet decrease and CSF cell count (r=0.63, p<0.005, Fig. 4).

Table 3 . CSF cell count in herpes zoster

	Total	Trigeminal lesion	p*	Spinal lesion	with Dissemination	p**	without Dissemination
Patients with pleocytosis (%)	49	50		48	67		44
Mean ± SD (/3)	167±237	207±297	(NS)	144±200	334±341	(<0.05)	111±165

* Probability between patients with trigeminal lesion and those with spinal lesion
** Probability between patients with and without dissemination

CSF cell count (/3)

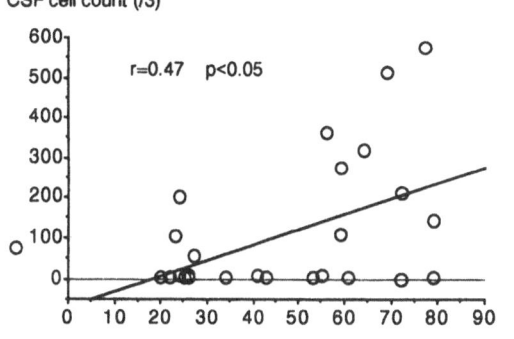

Fig. 3
Correlation between the age and CSF cell count in the patients without dissemination

CSF cell count (/3)

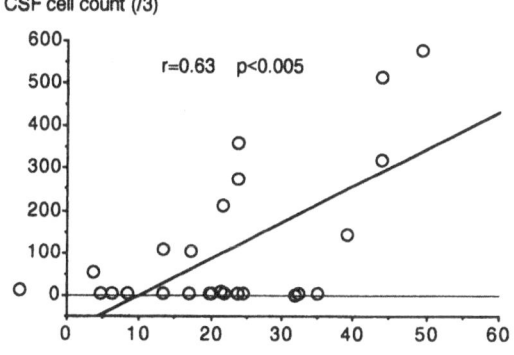

Fig. 4
Correlation between platelet decrease and CSF cell count in the patients without dissemination

DISCUSSION

The mechanism of involvement of central nervous system (CNS) in HZ has been well documented. It is summarized that (i) virus particles of VZV spread to ganglia, nerve fibers and CNS target nuclei via neurons; (ii) VZV hematogenously spread to microvessels in CNS and brainstem. Both neural and hematogenous pathways are considered to induce encephalitis [2]. However no intensive studies have been done as to hemostatic and fibrinolytic modulation in HZ, although studies of herpes simplex virus (HSV) infection indicated that anticoagulant properties of endothelial cells were shifted to procoagulant after HSV infection by prothrombinase complex formation and by increasing platelet binding [4]. The present results revealing significant platelet decrease may be interpreted by a similar mechanism. Earlier histopathological examination of herpetic lesion revealed that VZV is detected in damaging endothelial cells [2,3]. Such endothelial cell change may account for the present finding. In the present study, we observed that patients of HZ with dissemination, namely patients with viable VZV particles in the systemic circulation showed more abnormal change than those without dissemination.

It has been reported that thrombotic condition physiologically increases with age [5,6]. The present study demonstrating that more abnormal hemostatic change was observed in older patients was compatible to the physiologic change. We here additionally suggest that hemostatic and fibrinolytic risky condition is also in the patients younger than 40 years old, as well as the aged patients in VZV infection. It was reported that incidence of thrombotic disease increases in elderly females especially postmenopausal females [7]. In this study, however no difference was observed between male and female patients over 60 years old.

In addition the present study demonstrated that CSF pleocytosis in HZ is also correlated to the age of patients. This finding may account for the present observation that encephalitis after HZ increases in older patients [8]. Furthermore we would like to emphasize that the degree of hemostatic change is correlated to change in CSF. Monitoring precisely hematological parameters is suggested to be significantly important not only to detect risk of DIC but also to suggest increasing risk of CNS involvement.

REFERENCES
[1] Mckey DG, Margaretten W (1967) Arch Intern Med 120: 129-152
[2] Schmidbauer M, Budka H, Pilz P, Kurata T, Hondo R (1992) Brain 115: 383-398
[3] Muraki R, Baba T, Iwasaki T, Sata T, Kurata T (1992) Virchows Arch A Pathol Anat Histopathol 420: 71-76
[4] Visser MR, Tracy PB, Vercellotti GM, Goodman JL, White JG, Jacob HS (1988) Proc Natl Acad Sci USA 85: 8227-8230
[5] Hashimoto Y, Kobayashi A, Yamazaki N, Sugawara Y, Takada Y, Takada A (1987) Thromb Res 46: 625-633
[6] Takada Y, Takada A (1989) Thromb Res 55: 601-609
[7] Kannel WB, Hjortland MC, Mcnamara PM, Gordon T (1976) Ann Int Med 85: 447-452
[8] Gilden DH, Vafai A (1989) In: Vinken PJ, Bruyn GW, Klawans HL (eds) Handbook of Clinical Neurology Vol 56. Elsevier. Amsterdam. pp229-247

STUDY ON HYPERACTIVATED STATE OF COAGULATION AND FIBRINOLYSIS

K. DEGUCHI[1], T. TSUKADA[2], K. OONISHI[2], S. MURASHIMA[2], M. NISHIKAWA[2]

[1]Collage of Medical Science, [2]Second Department of Internal Medicine, Mie University Faculty of Medicine, Tsu city, Mie 514, Japan

INTRODUCTION

The excessive and untimely formation of blood clot(thrombus) in blood vessels may discontinue the blood supply to vital organ, and sometimes be followed by the aggravation of diseased state and the danger of life. The word "hypercoagulability" is often taken to mean an increased tendency to thrombose, and is usually used to mean an excess or activation of, clotting factors. Furthermore, as analogous words, prethrombotic state seem to imply the previous state of thrombosis, and prethrombotic state is used to connote a predisposition to thrombose(1). It is very important for the prophylaxis of overt thrombosis to know the behaviors of clotting and fibrinolytic factors in these state.

Recently, the development of the methods to determine the quantity of very small amounts of proteins enable us to detect the changes of coagulation and fibrinolysis system in the process of thrombosis formation. Such proteins are generally called molecular markers for coagulation or fibrinolysis, and were released or generated in the process of activation of clotting and/or fibrinolytic factors.

Plasma values of molecular markers for coagulation and fibrinolysis in various diseases were investigated to evaluate the information on foreknowledge and prophylaxis of the development of overt DIC and thrombosis.

MATERIALS and METHODS

Patients were divided into Type 1 group(65 leukemic patients, 315 samples) and Type II group(150 non-leukemic patients, 415 samples), according to the criteria proposed by the research committee on DIC of the Ministry of Health and Welfare in Japan(2), as previous reported(3), Blood was collected by venepuncture, and anticoagulated with 3.8% sodium citrate. Plasma was obtained by centrifugation for 15 min at 3,600g and $4^{\circ}C$, and stored at $-70^{\circ}C$. $Fragment_{1+2}$(F_{1+2}; ELISA, Behringwerke AG, Germany), thrombin/antithrombin III complex(TAT; ELISA, Behringwerke AG), plasmin/$alpha_2$ plasmin inhibitor complex(PIC; ELISA, Teijin Co., Japan), fibrin(ogen) degradation products(FDP; Latex aggregation method, Iatron Co., Japan), D-dimer(Latex aggregation method, Iatron Co.), tPA/PAI complex(TPAC; ELISA, Teijin Co., Japan), and thrombomodulin(TM; ELISA, Mitsubishi Gas Co., Japan) were measured.

RESULTS

1) A criteria of hyperactivated state of coagulation and/or fibrinolysis

The mean value ± 2SD(95% confidence interval) from 60 healthy subjects is 0.9-4.5 ng/ml in TAT, 0.14-1.02 nmol/L in F_{1+2}, 0-0.8 μg/ml in PIC, under 0.5 μg/ml in D-dimer, 4.5-18.3 ng/ml in TPAC, and 8.1-24.5 ng/ml in TM. In this study, the plasma values of molecular markers within their confidence interval were estimated as normal range.

A criteria was provided for diagnosis of hyperactivated state of coagulation and/or fibrinolysis. The criteria is that the values of plural molecular markers exceed simultaneously their upper limit of normal range; TAT$\geq$5.0, $F_{1+2}\geq$1.1, D-dimer$\geq$1.0 for coagulation, PIC$\geq$1.0, D-dimer$\geq$1.0 for fibrinolysis, and TAT$\geq$5.0, $F_{1+2}\geq$1.1, PIC$\geq$1.0, D-dimer$\geq$1.0 for coagulation and fibrinolysis.

2) Plasma values of molecular markers and the hyperactivated state of coagulation and fibrinolysis in various diseases

Fig. 1 show the mean plasma values of them from patients in Type I and II groups. The plasma value of each molecular marker varied in the degree among patients. High

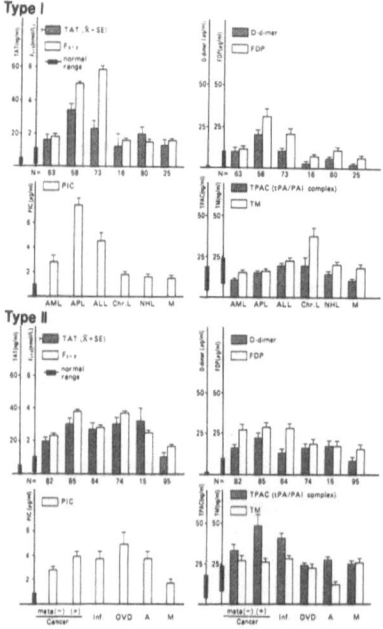

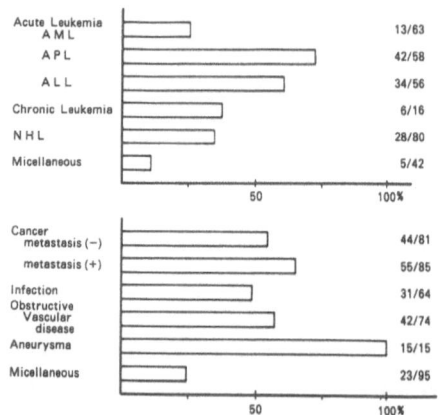

Fig. 2. Hyperactivated state of coagulation and fibrinolysis.

Fig. 1. Plasma values of molecular markers in various diseases. meta: metastasis, Inf.:infection, OVD: obstructive vascular disease, A: aneurysma, M: miscellaneous.

values of markers were observed in samples which were collected at the time of aggravation of diseased state, chemotherapy and blood transfusion. The mean values of TAT, F_{1+2}, PIC and D-dimer exceeded the upper limit of their normal range in Type I and II group, especially, acute leukemia, cancer, infection, obstructive vascular diseases and aneurysma. APL, ALL and diseases in Type II group showed higher mean value in FDP than normal range. The mean values of TM from diseases in Type II group and chronic leukemia were higher as compared with normal range.

All disease groups which were classified as shown in Fig. 2, were revealed to include the samples from patients with the hyperactivated state of coagulation and/or fibrinolysis. The incidence of samples from patients with the hyperactivated state of coagulation, fibrinolysis, and coagulation and fibrinolysis was 42.9, 50.8 and 40.6% in Type I group, 57.0, 68.8 and 50.7% in Type II group, respectively.

Fifty percent and overt of samples from patients with APL, ALL, cancer or obstructive vascular disease, and all samples from patients with aneurysma showed the hyperactivated state of coagulation and fibrinolysis.

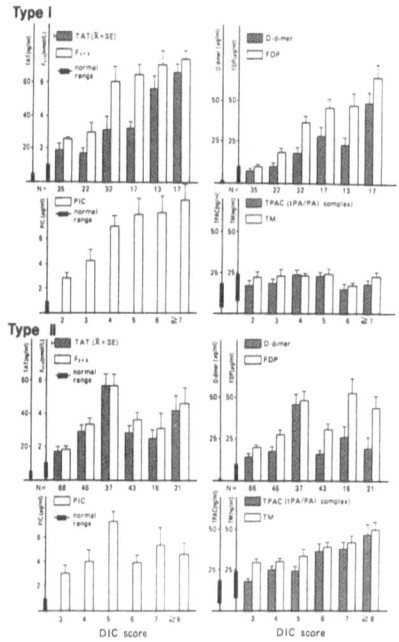

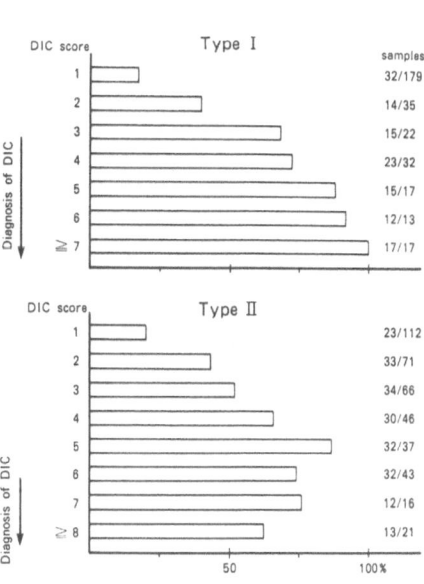

Fig. 3. Plasma values of molecular markers in each DIC score.

Fig. 4. Incidence of hyperactivated state of coagulation and fibrinolysis in each DIC score.

3) Plasma values of molecular markers and the hyperactivated state of coagulation and fibrinolysis in each DIC score

In type I group(Fig. 3), plasma mean values of TAT, F_{1+2}, PIC, D-dimer and FDP were higher than normal range and increased together with the grade of DIC score. But those of TPAC and TM in each DIC score were within their normal range. While, in Type II group(Fig. 3), plasma mean values of TAT, F_{1+2}, PIC and D-dimer increased in the order of DIC score 3, 4, 5 points and showed lower values in 6, 7, and over 8 than in 5 points. And the mean values of TPAC and TM increased together with the grade of DIC score.

Thirty-two of 179 samples in Type I group and 23 of 112 samples in Type II group showed the hyperactivated state of coagulation and fibrinolysis in spite of one point of DIC score. The incidence of samples of coagulation and fibrinolysis increased with the grade of DIC score in Type I group, and in the order of score 1,2,3,4 and 5 points in Type II group(Fig. 4).

DISCUSSION

In this study, the activation of clotting and fibrinolytic factors in blood circulation were revealed by the investigation of plasma concentration of molecular markers for coagulation and fibrinolysis in various diseases. High values of markers were observed in samples which were collected at the time of aggravation of diseased state, chemotherapy and blood transfusion. Therefore, plasma concentration of markers may be influenced by the aggravation of diseased state, and the treatment. The clotting and fibrinolytic factors were well known to be activated by activators such as tissue factor and cytokines released from monocyte, tumor cells and vascular endothelial cell, or on the damaged vascular surface(4,5,6,7). The molecular markers were released or generated in the process of activation of clotting and/or fibrinolytic factors. So, plasma concentration of molecular markers reflect the activated state of those factors. The releases of tissue factor and cytokines, and the damaged vascular surface may play important role on the elevation of plasma values of TAT, F_{1+2}, PIC and D-dimer in many of patients with acute leukemia, cancer, infection, obstructive vascular diseases or aneurysma.

A criteria was provided for diagnosis of the hyperactivated state of coagulation and/or fibrinolysis to simplify the information on the development of overt DIC and thrombosis. The criteria is that the values of plural molecular markers exceed simultaneously their upper limit of normal range. There are few papers on the estimation of coagulation and fibrinolysis from plasma value of plural molecular markers in the same specimen. The incidence of samples from patients with hyperactivated state of coagulation and fibrinolysis was higher in Type II group than Type I group. The incidence of such samples in disease groups was dependent on the degree of mean plasma values of markers.

DIC score proposed by the research committee on DIC of the Ministry of Health and Welfare in Japan is mainly estimated from the degree of consumption of clotting factors and platelets(2). As shown in Fig. 3 and 4, Type II group differed from Type I group in the mean values of markers and the incidence of samples from patients with hyperactivated state of coagulation and fibrinolysis in each DIC score. This may arise from the difference between Type I group and Type II group in the progress of DIC and in the management for basic diseases. DIC in Type I group develops almost rapidly, and are treated with sufficient blood transfusion as well as chemotherapy for basic disease. While, many of DIC in Type II group develop more slowly than in Type I group. The mean values of markers from Type II group in each DIC score suggested that a diagnosis of DIC according to the criteria for DIC has been done after the stage of intensive activation of clotting and fibrinolytic factors in circulating blood.

In conclusion, plasma values of TAT, F_{1+2}, PIC and D-dimer inform us on the stage of activation of clotting and/or fibrinolytic factors, and enable us to diagnose the hyperactivated state of coagulation and fibrinolysis in circulation blood. Therefore, those markers may be available to evaluate the information on foreknowledge and prophylaxis of the development of overt DIC and thrombosis.

REFERENCES

1. O'Brien JR, Ed by Poller L. (1977) Recent advance in blood coagulation. Churchill Livingstone. Edinburgh, London and New York. pp241-266

2. Aoki N, Hasegawa H, Ed by Aoki N (1988) Annual report of the Research Committee on Coagulation Disorder. Ministry of Health and Welfare of Japan. Tokyo. pp37-41

3. Deguchi K, Noguchi M, Yuwasaki E, Endou T, Deguchi A, Wada H, Murashima S, Nishikawa M, Shirakawa S, Tanaka K, Kusagawa M (1991) Am J Hematol 38: 86-89

4. Gralnick HR, Abrell E (1973) Br J Haematol24: 89

5. Bauer KA, Rosenberg RD (1984) Blood 64: 791

6. Cozzolino F, Torcia M, Miliani A, Carossino AM, Giordani R, Cinotti S, Filimberti E, Saccardi R, Bernablei P, Guidi G, DiGuglielmo R, Pistoia V, Ferrarini M, Nawroth PP,Stern D (1988) Am J Med 84: 240

7. Nawroth PP, Hanley D, Esmon CT, Stern DM (1986) Proc Natl Acad Sci USA 83: 3460

Flow cytometric analysis of tumor-associated proteases with special reference to uPA/PAI-1 complex

N. MONIWA, T. TERAO [1], N. CHUCHOLOWSKI, M. SCHMITT, and H. GRAEFF [2]

[1] Department of Obstetrics and Gynecology, Hamamatsu University School of Medicine, 3600 Handa-cho, Hamamatsu, 431-31, Japan
[2] Frauenklinik der Technischen Universitat München, Ismaninger Str. 22, 8000 München 80, FRG

Key words: urokinase type plasminogen activator/plasminogen activator inhibitor type 1(uPA/PAI-1) complex, cell proliferation, flow cytometry(FCM), internalization of urokinase type plasminogen activator receptor(uPAR)

Introduction

There is evidence that in invasion and metastasis of solid tumors tumor-associated proteases are involved in dissolution of the surrounding tomor matrix and the basement membranes. A key role of urokinase type plasminogen activator(uPA)-mediated proteolysis was demonstrated by a series of experiments showing that inhibition of uPA activity blocks metastasis or invasion [8, 9]. uPA converts plasminogen to plasmin and thus mediates pericellular proteolysis during cell migration and tissue remodelling under physiological and pathophysiological conditions. uPA exerts its proteolytic function on normal cells and tumor cells as an ectoenzyme after its binding to a high-affinity cell surface receptor(uPAR).

Tissues of primary cancers and/or metastases of the breast[1, 5], ovary, prostate, cervix uteri, bladder, lung and gastro-intenstinal tract have higher levels of uPA than benign tumors. Consistent with these findings, patients with tumors having relatively high pro-uPA/uPA contents show significantly shorter relapse-free survival and shorter overall survival than patients with tumors having lower pro-uPA/uPA levels. The clinical course of breast cancer is associated not only with a high uPA content but also with an increased level of plasminogen activator inhibitor type 1(PAI-1), which is a specific plasminogen inhibitor[5]. Moreover, the relapse rate of patients in which the primary tumors have high PAI-1 antigen contents is significantly more than that of patients in which the primary tumor have low PAI-1 contents[4]. These findings somewhat contradictory since a high level of the inhibitor should block the enzymatic activity of receptor-bound uPA.

Recently, it was found that receptor-bound uPA and pro-uPA are not internalized or degraded, but that enzymatically inactive uPA/PAI complexes are internalized and degraded. Thus cells are able to regulate not only the amount, but also the location of cell surface uPA activity [3, 4]. This would explain how the location of uPA activity determines the direction of proteolysis in cellular migration and invasion.

We studied the rapid and quantitative change of cell surface receptors and antigens of single cells by flow cytometry(FCM)[2]. Here we report studies on the internalization of the uPAR binding uPA/PAI-1 complex. We found that its internalization is closely related with the proliferation of tumor cells.

MATERIALS AND METHODS

Recombinant human PAI-1 and mouse monoclonal antibodies(MAb) #377 to human u-PA, #3783 to human melanoma PAI-1 and #3936 to human uPAR were obtained from American Diagnostica(Greenwitch, CT). HMW-uPA[urokinase], active two-chain high-molecular-weight form of uPA, was purchased from Ribosepharm(Haan, FRG). 5-

Bromo-2'-deoxyuridine (BrdU), propidium iodide(PI) and FITC-conjugated goat-anti-mouse-IgG were purchased from Sigma(München, FRG). Monoclonal anti-BrdU antibody were purchased from Becton Dickinson(Heidelberg, FRG). HMW-uPA conjugated FITC was prepared in our laboratory.

Cells and cell culture

Cells of the histiocytic lymphoma cell line U937, which have monocyte-like characteristics, were grown in RPMI 1640 supplemented with 10 % fetal calf serum(GIBCO, Eggestein, FRG), 2.5 μg of amphotericin B / ml and 0.1 mg gentamycin / ml(BIOCHROM, Berlin, FRG). Differentiated (stimulated) U937 cells were obtained by incubation in above medium containing 1 μM phorbol-12-myristate-13-acetate 4-0-metyl ether(PMA, Sigma). A 3-day incubation with Hank's buffer standard solution(HBSS), harvested by centrifugation and resuspended in HBSS.

Immunofluorescence to cell surface antigens

Unstimulated or PMA-stimulated U937 cells(1×10^6) were incubated with #3689, #3783 or #3936 antibody at RT for 30 min. After centrifugation(300 $\times$ g, 10min, 22° C) and washed twice, resuspended in 250 μl of HBSS, pH 7.4, and incubated with 4 μl of anti-mouse IgG FITC for 30 min at RT. They were then centrifuged(300 $\times$ g, 10min, 22° C) and washed twice, the cell-associated fluorescence was quantified by flow cytometry.

Receptor-mediated internalization of bound HMW-uPA with PAI-1

Unstimulated or PMA-stimulated U937 cells(1×10^6) were transferred from culture medium to 0.5 ml of a solution of 50 mM glycine-HCl pH 3.0, containing 0.1M NaCl, for 1 min at 22 ° C to dissociate receptor-bound uPA. Then the buffer was neutralized by addition of 0.5 ml of 0.5 M HEPES-buffer pH 7.5, containing 0.1 M NaCl. The cells were collected by centrifugation(300 $\times$ g, 10min, 22° C), washed twice, resuspended in 500μl ofHBSS, pH 7.4, and incubated with 10 nM HMW-UPA FITC for 30 min at RT. After washed twice, they were then incubated in the absence or presence of 1μM PAI-1 at 37 ° C. After one wash with HBSS, their cell-associated fluorescence was quantified by flow cytometory. Then 1.5 ml of 50 mM glycine-HCl pH 3.0, containing 0.1M NaCl, was promptly added, and their fluorescence wwas measured again.

Cell cycle analysis by double staining with BrdU and PI

Samples of 1×10^6 cells were incubated with 15μM BrdU for 30 min at 37 ° C in a 5% CO_2 incubator, and washed twice with PBS. The cells were then resuspended in 600μl of PBS and 1400 μl of cold absolute ethanol were added with vortexing(70 % ethanol fixation). The cells were stored overnight in 4 ° C, and then washed twice with PBS, resuspended in 2 ml of 2N HCl containing 0.5 mg of Pepsin(Sigma), incubated for 30 min at RT. They were then washed twice with PBS, resuspended in 7 ml of 0.5 M Hepes buffer(pH 7.5). They were washed twice with PBS, resuspended in 1 ml of PBS containing 0.5 % Tween 20 and 0.5 % BSA, and incubated for 30 min at RT with 20 μl of anti BrdU. After two buffers washs with PBS, they were resuspended in 1 ml of PBS including 0.5 % Tween 20 and 0.5 % BSA, and incubated for 30 min at RT with 4μl of anti mouse IgG FITC. After washed twice in PBS, cells were resuspended in 500μl of PBS containing 0.5 mg of RNase(Sigma) and incubated for 30 min at RT. Finally, 5 μl of 1 mg/ml PI solution was added, and the cells were incubated for 20 min at RT. Flow cytometric analysis was perfomed within 1h.

Flow cytometry(FCM)

FCM analysis was performed with a standard FACScan instrument(Becton Dickinson, Heidelberg, FRG) with an air-cooled Argon ion laser emitting 15mW at 488nm. The instrument was equipped with two fluorescence detector photomultiplier tubes, green fluorescence(FITC) being collected through a 530/80 nm bandpass, and red fluorescence(PI) through a 650 nm long pass filter. Both linear and logarithmic amplifiers were used to process the fluorescence of antibodies. The data of 10-20,000 events were collected, stored in a list mode and analyzed using Consort 30 software.

RESULTS

Effect of PMA stimulation of U937 cells

We measured the fluorescence intensity(FI) of cellular surface antigens after incubation of cells for 3 days with or without PMA(Fig. 1A, 1B, 1C). The fluorescence intensity of the surface of PMA-stimulated cells was higher than that of unstimulated cells, indicating that PMA-stimulated cells had higher levels of surface antigen than unstimulated cells. FI of the uPAR was especially increased about 30-fold, wheras that of uPA was increased only about 2.4-fold and that to PAI-1 was increased about 1.7-fold.

Receptor-mediated internalization of HMW-uPA bound with PAI-1

The uPA/PAI-1 complex was formed during incubation of uPA with a 10-fold molar excess of PAI-1 at RT for 15 min(data not shown).

First we studied whether cells stimulated with PMA which had many receptors(Fig. 1B), had the capacity to internalize uPAR. Cells preincubated with HMW-uPA and cells preincubated with HMW-uPA plus PAI-1 both showed decreased FI of uPAR binding FITC-conjugated HMW-uPA, but no change of intracellular FI(Fig. 2A, 2B). Thus these cells had no ability to internalize uPAR.

Next we examined whether cells without PMA stimulation had any capacity to internalize uPAR. Cells preincubated with HMW-uPA had no capacity to internalize uPAR(Fig. 3A). But cells preincubated with HMW-uPA plus PAI-1(cellular surface uPA-R binding uPA/PAI-1 complex) showed decrease of FI of cell surface uPAR and increase of FI of intracellular FITC during incubation for 3 hours. Thus the uPAR binding the uPA/PAI-1 complex was internalized(Fig. 3B). We suppose that internalization of uPAR occurred in unstimulated U937 cells.

Internalization of uPAR and celluar proliferation

We found that cells in which uPAR was internalized showed morphological transformation(data not shown). First, we analysed the cell cycle using FCM with single color staining with PI(Fig. 4A). But by this method, we did not obtain clear separation of cells at different stages of the cell cycles, the early S-phase overlappe the G0/G1-phase and the late S-phase overlapping the G2/M-phase(data not shown). Therefore, we used double color staining with FITC and PI. And in this way obtained clear separation of different stages of the cell cycle(Fig. 4B). Three groups of cells were prepared: 1)cells, 2)cells preincubated with HMW-uPA, and 3)cells preincubated with HMW-uPA and PAI-1. Cells was incubated for 24 hours under 5% CO_2 , and analysed the cells at intervals(Fig. 5). Results showed that the cell cycles changed after 6-hours incubation. In groups 1 and 2, cells accumulated in the G0/G1-phase with gradual decrease of cells in the S-phase. In contrast, in group 3, cells in the S-phase clearly increased with decrease of cells in the G0/G1-phase from 6 to 15 hours of incubation. These findings indicate that internalization of the uPAR binding HMW-uPA/PAI-1 complex transmitted a signal to the cytoplasm or directly to the nucleus leading to cell proliferation.

DISCUSSION

Flow cytometry has been widly used to detect and quantify surface antigens, including receptors. Functional uPA-R on living cells has been quantified using FITC-HMW-uPA as a specific ligand. The antigen specificities of the respective antibodies were assessed using established tumor cell lines[2] .

Previously, the celular characteristics of U937 cells, a human monocyte-like cell line, were found to change on chemotaxis like PMA stimulation, PMA-stimulated cells having higher contents of ·uPA and uPAR than cells without PMA-stimulation. We found that the number of uPAR was remarkedly increased and hat cell surface antigens of uPA and PAI-1 also increased;there is a problem of whether U937 cells actually produce PAI-1[6] .

The uPA content of tumors is closely related with the prognosis of patients with malignant tumors and at first supposing that PMA-stimulated cells had the capacity to internalize uPAR. We wondered why they had a high content of uPA. But we found that the uPAR of PMA stimulated cells could not be internalized. This means that PMA stimulated cells have a large number of uPAR but that the uPAR may be dysfunctional or only supply uPA at their site on the surface.

The internalization of uPAR binding the uPA/PAI-1 complex was previously demonstrated by fluorescence microscopy and autoradiography[3, 4] . In the present study we demonstrated using FCM that uPAR binding HMW-uPA/PAI-1 complex on U937 cells could be internalized. The total fluorescence mean channel(FMC) was stable, and FMC associated with the cell surface decreasing gradually. This means that intracellular FMC graduatly increased, namely internalization occured. The uPAR binding the HMW-uPA/PAI-1 complex on U937 cells only could be internalized but the uPAR binding HMW-uPA could not.

Why is uPAR on tumor cells internalized? If uPAR can be internalized and degraded only when complexed with PAI, we thought that this would result in self-inhibition of cell growth. We found in this study that the cell size was increased the intracellular struction of the cells changed after internalizatio n of the uPAR binding uPA/PAI-1 complex(the cell size and intracellular struction can be measured by forward scatter and side scatter of FCM). This result suggested that tumor cells may be stimulated by uPAR internalization. There are clinical reports that patients with high levels of PAI-1 have a poor prognosis. Jänicke et al. reported that patients with high PAI-1 levels have a significant higher relapse rate than those with low PAI-1 levels and that there is a significant correlation between S-phase values and'PAI-1 levels in primary breast cancer[5] . Furthermore, in vitro experiments have shown that some cells that produced high levels of uPA were poorly invasive under standard conditions but invasion was enhanced by PAI[7] . These results seem somewhat contradictory since high levels of the inhibitor should be protective by blocking the enzymatic activity of receptor-bound uPA. However, We found that U937 cells showed increased proliferative activity(an increased frequency of S-phase cells) after internalization of uPAR binding the uPA/PAI-1 complex. This means that excess release of PAI-1 into tumor tissue may be of importance for the process of metastasis, that is reimplantation of circulating tumor cells into tissues after their release from the primary site.'Though uPA activity is depressed by the action of PAI-1, generation and growth of metastases may be supported by the signal of internalization. Internalization of the receptor binding the uPA/PAI-1 complex in tumor cells may also be the trigger for cell proliferation.

REFFERENCES
1. Jänicke F., Schmitt M., Hafter R., Hollrieder A., Babic R., Ulm K., Gössner W. and Graeff H.(1990) Fibrinolysis 4,69-78
2. Chucholowski N., Schmitt, M., Goretzki L., Schüren E., Moniwa N., Weidle U., Kramer M., Wagner B., Jänicke F. and Graeff H.(1992) Biochemical Society Transactions 20, 208-216
3. Olson D., Pöllänen J., Hoyer-Hansen G., Ronne E., Sakaguchi K., Wun T-C., Appella E., Dano K. and Blasi F.(1992) J. Bioe. Chem. 267, 9129-9133

4. Cubellis MV., Wun T-C., Blasi F.(1990) EMBO J. 9, 1079-1084
5. Jänicke F., Schmiitt M. and Greaff H.(1991) Sem. Thromb. Hem. 17, 303-312
6. Cajot J-F., Kruithof E., Schleuning W-D., Sordat B. and Bachmann F.(1986) Int. J. Cancer 38, 719-727
7. Tuboi R. and Rifkin DB(1990) Int. J. Cancer 46, 56-60
8. Ossowski l. and Reich E.(1983) Cell 35, 611-619
9. Hearing V.J., Law L.W., Corti A., Apella E. and Blasi F.(1988) Cancer Res. 48, 1270-1278

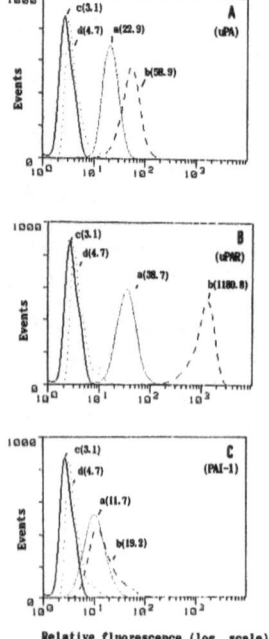

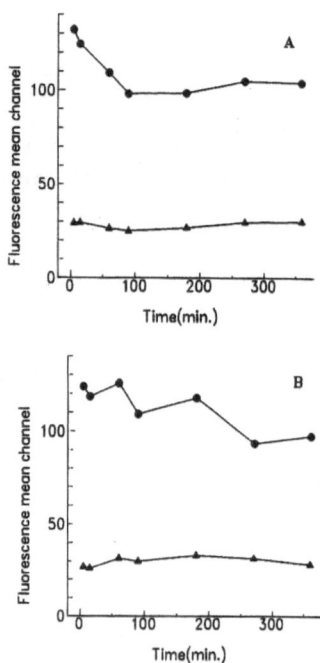

Fig. 1 Detection of the proteases uPA, the receptors for urokinase(uPAR) and the uPA-inhibitor PAI-1 in U937 cells by flow cytometry(FCM) applying monoclonal antibodies. Designation of the lines is as follows; Line A: unstimulated U937 cells + monoclonal antibody and mouse IgG FITC. Line B: PMA stimulated U937 cells + monoclonal antibody and mouse IgG FITC. Line C: unstimulated U937 cells + mouse IgG FITC(control). Line B: PMA stimulated U937 cells + mouse IgG FITC(control). ( ) is discribed fluorescence mean channel.

Fig. 2 Internalization of uPAR receptors binding FITC-HMW-uPA with/without PAI-1 on PMA stimulated U937 cells depend on time of incubation. (A) PMA stimulated U937 cells with FITC HMW-uPA. (B) PMA stimulated U937 cells with FITC HMW-uPA + PAI-1. ●: total fluorescence mean channnel(FMC) ▲: intracelluar FMC.

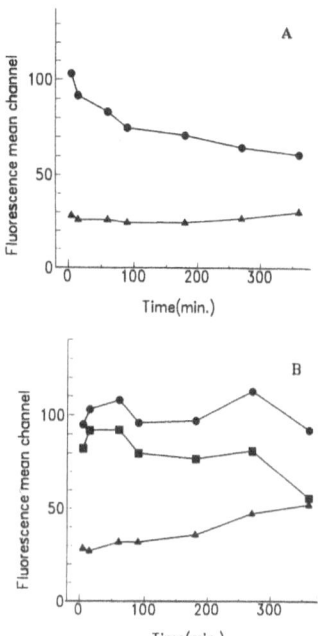

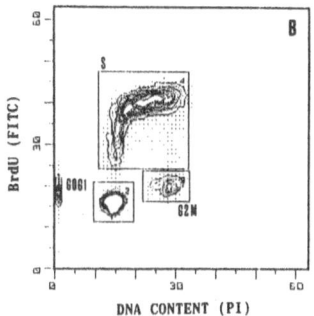

Fig. 3 Internalization of uPAR receptors binding
FITC-HMW-uPA with/without PAI-1 on unstimulated
U937 cells depend on time of incubation. (A)
unstimulated U937 cells with FITC HMW-uPA. (B)
unstimulated U937 cells with FITC HMW-uPA + PAI-1.
●: total fluorescence mean channnel(FMC) ▲:
intracelluar FMC ■: cell surface FMC[total FMC
- intracelluar FMC + blank FMC].

Fig. 4 Cell cycle analysis on U937 cells by using
flow cytometry. (A) single color staining of PI.
(B) double color staining of PI and FITC(BrdU).

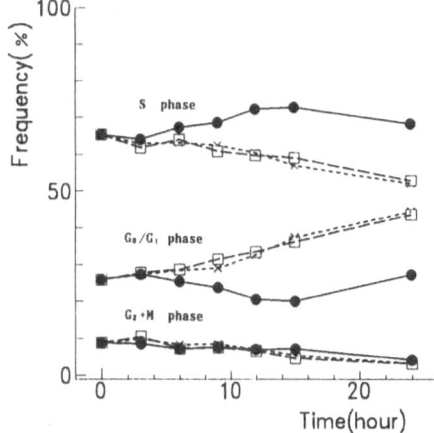

Fig. 5 The relationship between uPAR receptors
binding FITC-HMW-uPA with/without PAI-1 and cell
cycle analysis on unstimulated U937 cells depend
on time of incubation. ✕: unstimulated U937
cells □: unstimulated U937 cells with 10 nM of
HMW-uPA ●: unstimulated U937 cells with 10 nM of
HMW-uPA and 1 μM of PAI-1.

RELATIONSHIPS BETWEEN THE CONCENTRATIONS OF u-PA, t-PA, PAI-1 and PAI-2 IN TUMOR TISSUES AND PERITONEAL WASHINGS, AND TUMOR PROGRESSION IN GASTRIC CANCER

N. NISHINO[1], M. NAKAMURA[1], H. KONNO[1], S. BABA[1], K. AOKI[2], O. YONEKAWA[3], E. HAMADA[3], T. KANNO[3], S. TAKAHASHI[4], M. CHO[4], T. URANO[4], Y. TAKADA[4] AND A. TAKADA[4]

[1]Departments of Surgery, [2]Emergency Medicine, [3]Laboratory Medicine, and [4]Physiology, Hamamatsu University School of Medicine, Shizuoka, Japan.

SUMMARY

The concentrations of u-PA, t-PA, PAI-1 and PAI-2 in tumor extracts and in peritoneal washings from patients with gastric cancer were examined, and relationships between these parameters and a progression of the gastric cancer were evaluated. The levels of u-PA, PAI-1 and PAI-2 were higher in cancer than in control tissues, whereas levels of t-PA were not different between tumor tissue and adjacent mucosa. No difference was observed in tissue levels of u-PA among various extents of lymph node involvement. However, PAI-1 levels in the primary cancer tissues tended to increase when cancer cells metastasized to remote lymph node. PAI-2 levels tended to decrease when more distant lymphatic metastasis was present, indicating that lower levels of PAI-2 in the primary cancer tissue may make it possible to develop metastasis. The levels of u-PA and PAI-2 in peritoneal washings did not correlate with the depth of cancer invasion. However, the levels of t-PA and PAI-1 significantly increased as the depth of cancer invasion progressed. These results indicate that the groups with the low levels of PAI-2 in cancer tissues and the high levels of t-PA and PAI-1 in peritoneal washings are thought to be groups with high possibility of metastasis in gastric cancer.

KEYWORDS : gastric cancer, metastasis, plasminogen activator, plasminogen activator inhibitor

INTRODUCTION

Recently, much attention has been paid to roles of plasminogen activator (PA) and plasminogen activator inhibitor (PAI) in tumor growth and the mechanisms of metastasis(1-5). Urinary type PA (u-PA) has recently been reported to be produced mainly from fibroblast in tumor tissues(6). u-PA derived from fibroblast binds to its specific receptor of tumor cell surface, results in the activated form of u-PA. Once the u-PAs are activated they convert plasminogen to plasmin in most extracellular tissues. In that way u-PA may participate in the normal and pathological modulation of extracellular matrix, since in addition to being fibrinolytic, plasmin can degrade noncollagenous matrix component such as laminin and fibronectin(1,7). t-PA is supposed to be localized to the vascular endothelium of many tissues and be a key enzyme in thrombolysis(8). The role of t-PA in the regulation of tumor growth and metastasis is less clear, or t-PA may have no role in these aspects. PAIs are specific inhibitors for PAs, and may play important roles in cancer tissues to control its growth and metastasis by regulating the activity of PAs(9).

We have measured the concentrations of u-PA, t-PA, PAI-1 and PAI-2 in tumor extracts and in peritoneal washings from patients with gastric cancer, and relationships between these parameters and a progression of gastric cancer were evaluated.

MATERIAL AND METHODS

Tissue extract samples
Tumor specimens were obtained from 50 patients who underwent the operation of gastric cancer in the Department of Surgery, Hamamatsu University Hospital. All specimens were examined microscopically, and the histrogical types and the number of lymph node involvements of each case were examined and recorded.

After surgery, the tissues were rinsed in saline to remove blood and fat. Then, the saline was removed with a filter paper, and the tissue frozen at -70 °C. The tissue was thawed, cut in pieces, put in 0.1 M Tris buffer containing 0.15 M NaCl, pH 7.4, and homogenized by 5 times repetition of 10 seconds' burst with 30 seconds' cooling interval in ice-water by microhomogenizer Physcotron (NITI-ON Tokyo Japan). The supernatant was taken and frozen till used.

Peritoneal washings
Peritoneal washings were obtained from 44 patients who underwent the operation of gastric cancer without ascites at laparotomy. Just after laparotomy, each 100 ml of saline was administered into left subphrenic space and Douglas' pouch and each 50 ml of saline samples was collected. After centrifugation at 3,000 rpm for 20 minutes, the surpernatant of each sample was concentrated approximately 50-fold with ultra filtration. The sample was frozen till used.

Elisa
u-PA and t-PA antigen levels were measured by enzyme immunoassay, previously reported from our laboratory (10,11). PAI-1 and PAI-2 antigen levels were measured by the enzyme linked immunosorbent assay kit (TintElize PAI-1 and TintElize PAI-2, Biopool Sweden). The measurement of the protein concentration of samples was performed by BIORAD Protein Assay kit (BIORAD, USA).

Classification of the depth of invasion of tumor and lymph node involvement
The extent of the depth of cancer infiltration to the gastric wall was classified according to the clinicopathological staging described in the General Rules of the Japanese Gastric Cancer Society(12). The depth of cancer infiltration was classified as 'm,sm', 'pm', 'ss', 'se' and 'sei,si'. Lymph nodal involvement was also classified as n0 to n3<, in which n0 has no detectable metastasis of cancer cells in regional lymph nodes. The n number indicates the grading of metastasis.

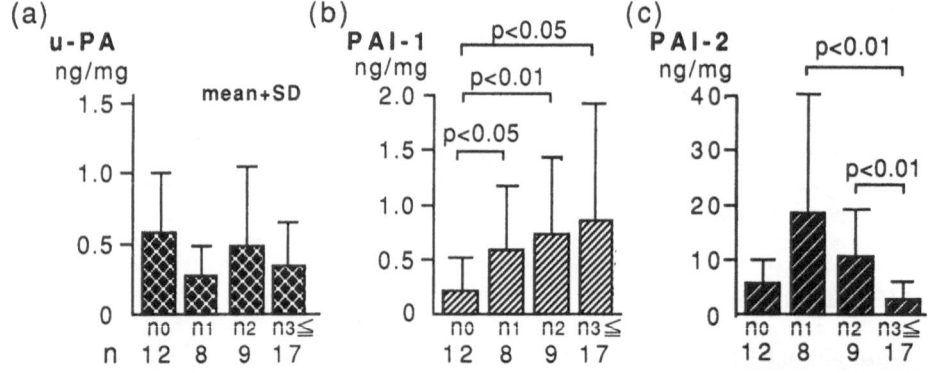

Fig.1 Relationships between the levels of u-PA, PAI-1 and PAI-2 in the primary tumor tissues, and lymph node involvement. n0 has no lymph nodal involvement, n3≦indicate the nodal involvement to the major draining lymph nodes. Numbers in the bottom indicate sample numbers.

Statistical analysis
    Students' t-test was used for significance.

RESULTS

Determination of u-PA, t-PA, PAI-1 and PAI-2 in cancer tissues and normal mucosa.
    The amounts of u-PA, t-PA, PAI-1 and PAI-2 antigens were determined in cancer tissues and their adjacent normal mucosa. The amounts of u-PA, PAI-1 and PAI-2 were significantly higher in cancer tissues than in adjacent mucosa. In contrast to these levels, the amounts of t-PA were not different between tumor tissues and adjacent mucosa. (Date not shown)

Relationships between tissue levels of u-PA, PAI-1 and PAI-2, and lymph node involvement
    The relationships between the concentrations of u-PA, PAI-1 and PAI-2 in the primary cancer tissue and the extent of metastasis to lymph nodes were examined. No difference was observed in the tissue levels of u-PA among various extents of lymph node involvement(Fig.1-a). However, PAI-1 levels in the primary cancer tissues tended to increase when cancer cells metastasized to remote lymph nodes. PAI-1 levels of n0 group, which had no lymphatic metastasis, were significantly lower than those of other groups(Fig.1-b). PAI-2 levels tended to decrease when more distant lymphatic metastasis was present. In the n3≦ group PAI-2 levels were significantly lower than in n1 or n2 group, indicating that lower levels of PAI-2 in the primary cancer tissue may be related to the development of metastasis(Fig.1-c).

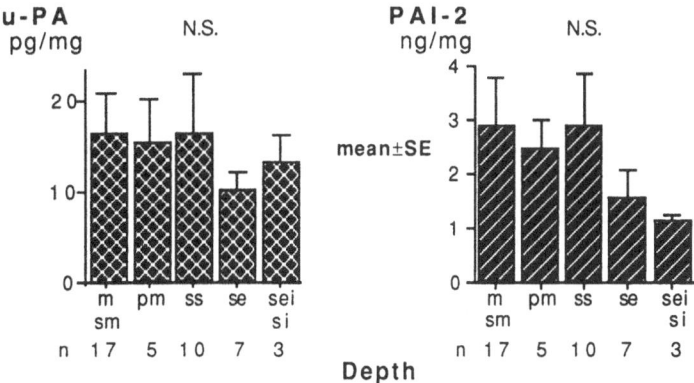

Fig.2 Relationships between the levels of u-PA and PAI-2 in the peritoneal washings, and the depth of invasion. m-si indicates the depth of invasion. m: mucosa, sm: submucosa, pm: proper muscle, ss: subserosa, se: serosa exposed, sei and si: invade to another organ. Numbers in the bottom indicate sample numbers.

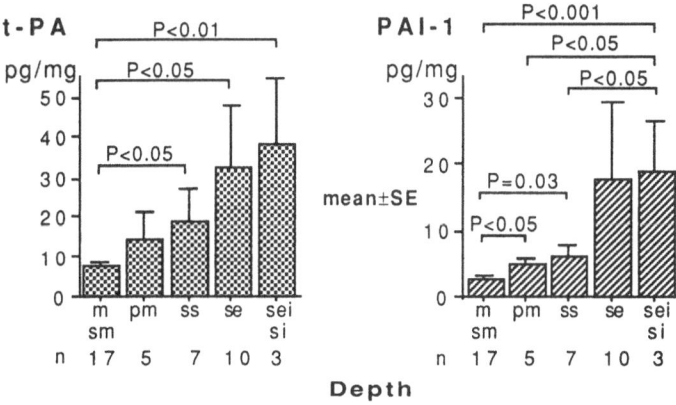

Fig.3 Relationships between the levels of t-PA and PAI-1 in the peritoneal washings, and the depth of invasion.

Relationships between levels of u-PA, t-PA, PAI-1 and PAI-2 in the peritoneal washings, and the depth of invasion

The relationship between the concentration of u-PA, t-PA, PAI-1 and PAI-2 in the peritoneal washings from patients with gastric cancer and the depth of cancer invasion were evaluated. The levels of u-PA and PAI-2 in peritoneal washings did not correlate with the depth of cancer invasion(Fig.2). However, the levels of t-PA and PAI-1 significantly increased as the depth of cancer invasion progressed(Fig.3).

DISCUSSION

Recently, many papers, which described the roles of plasminogen activator (PA) and plasminogen activator inhibitor (PAI) in tumor growth and the mechanisms of metastasis, have been reported(1-6). It is well known that u-PA is related to the regulations of tumor growth and metastasis(1,13). It is also known that PAIs are specific inhibitors for PAs, and may play important roles in cancer tissues to control its growth and metastasis by regulating the activity of PAs(9). In contrast, the role of t-PA in regulations of tumor growth and metastasis is less clear.

The post surgical prognosis of gastric cancer has been reported to be heavily influenced by the degree of tumor infiltration into the gastric wall and by the extent of lymph node metastasis(14). In gastric cancer the peritoneal recurrence is seen most frequently. This type of recurrence is considered to be caused by the exfoliation of cancer cells from the primary tumor which invaded into serosal surface. Moreover lymph nodal recurrence is also seen frequently.

In the present study we measured the concentrations of u-PA, t-PA, PAI-1 and PAI-2 in the primary tumor tissues and in the peritoneal washings from patients with gastric cancer, and the investigation whether or not levels of u-PA, t-PA, PAI-1 and PAI-2 were related to the extent of the invasion of the tumor and lymph nodal involvement was carried out. The reason why we used peritoneal washings as samples is to evaluate fibrinolytic activity, which is related to cancer, in the peritoneal cavity of patients with gastric cancer without ascites.

In this study we have shown that the antigen levels of u-PA, PAI-1 and PAI-2 in the primary gastric cancer tissues were higher than in the adjacent healthy gastric mucosa. When the extent of metastasis to lymph nodes was compared, primary tumor with higher PAI-1 levels tend to metastasize to more remote lymph nodes(Fig.1-b). On the other hand, PAI-2 levels were lower in primary tumor with more lymph node involvement (n3) than with less involvement (n1 or n2)(Fig.1-c). These results suggest that increase in PAI-2 levels results in the prevention of the spread and metastasis of gastric cancer, but PAI-1 rather increase with the growth or metastasis of the tumor.

Furthermore, we have shown the relationships between the concentrations of u-PA, t-PA, PAI-1 and PAI-2 in the peritoneal washings from patients with gastric cancer and the depth of cancer invasion. The levels of u-PA and PAI-2 in peritoneal washings did not correlate with the depth of cancer invasion(Fig.2). However, the levels of t-PA and PAI-1 significantly increased as the depth of cancer invasion progressed(Fig.3). As mentioned above, it is well known that u-PA is related to the regulation of tumor growth and metastasis, whereas t-PA is not thought to be related to their regulation. Huber et al. demonstrated in their study with ascites that no u-PA antigen could be detected in ascites of non-malignant and malignant origin. They showed that there was positive evidence for detectable tumor cells in peritoneal cavity in some of the patients with malignancies, and that malignant as well as non-malignant ascites contained appreciable amounts of t-PA. Thus, in their discussion they mentioned that the predominant PA type in ascites was not u-PA, but t-PA(15). In our study, not only t-PA antigen but also u-PA, PAI-1 and PAI-2 antigens were detected in peritoneal washings. In these parameters, the levels of u-PA and PAI-2 in peritoneal washings did not correlate with the depth of cancer invasion, whereas the levels of t-PA and PAI-1 significantly increased as the depth of cancer invasion progressed. From these results, PA related to malignancy in peritoneal cavity may be t-PA. It is unclear how t-PA levels increase as tumor progresses in peritoneal cavity. It may be a host reaction or a tumor specific phenomenon.

In conclusion, 1) increase in the levels of PAI-2, not PAI-1, in the primary tumor may prevent growth or development of metastasis of gastric cancer, 2) the groups with high levels of t-PA and PAI-1 in peritoneal washings are thought to be groups with high possibility of recurrence of gastric cancer.

REFERENCE

1. Tryggvason K, Hoyhtya M, Sato T (1987) Biochim Biophys Acta 907: 191-217
2. Nishino N, Aoki K, Tokura Y, Sakaguchi S, Takada Y, Takada A (1988) Thromb Res 50: 527-535
3. Nishino N, Nakamura M, Aoki K, Konno H, Baba S, Takada A (1991) Jpn J Gastroenterol Surg (Japanese abstract) 24(4) 1096-1100
4. Nakamura M, Konno H, Tanaka T, Maruo Y, Nishino N, Aoki K, Baba S, Sakaguchi S, Takada Y, Takada A (1992) Thromb Res 65: 709-719
5. Sappino AP, Busso N, Belin D, Vassali JD (1987) Cancer Res 47: 4043-4046
6. Pyke C, Kristensen P, Ralfkiaer E, Eriksen J, Dano K (1991) Cancer Res 51: 4067-4071
7. Skriver L, Nielsen LS, Stephens R, Dano K (1982) Eur J Biochem 124: 409-414
8. Kristensen P, Larsson LS, Nielsen LS, Grondahl-Hansen J, Andreasen PA, Dano K (1984) FEBS Lett 168: 33-37
9. Feinberg RF, Kao LC, Haimowitz JE, Queenan JT, Wun TC, Strauss III, Kliman HJ (1989) Labo Invest 61: 20-26
10. Takada Y, Shirahama S, Nagase M, Takada A (1985) J Clin Lab   Immunol 16: 169-172
11. Takada A, Shizume K, Ozawa T, Takahashi S, Takada Y (1986) Thromb Res 42:63-72
12. Japanese Research Society for Gastric Cancer: The General Rules for Gastric Cancer Study in Surgery and Pathology (1981) 11: 127-129
13. Dano K, Andreasen PA, Grondahl-Hansen J, Kristensen P, Nielsen IS, Skriver L (1985) Cancer Res 44: 140-240
14. Miwa K, and Japanese Research Society for Gastric Cancer (1984) Jpn J Clin Oncol 14(3): 385-410
15. Huber K, Wojta J, Kirchheimer C, Ermler D, Binder BR (1988) Eur J Clin Invest 18: 595-599

The Role of Hemodynamics in Atherogenesis

Kenji Sakakibara[1,2], Terue Sakakibara[1,3], Michael C.K. Chang[1] and Shu Chien[1]

Institute for Biomedical Engineering and Department of Applied Mechanics and Engineering Science[1], University of California, San Diego, La Jolla, California 92093-0412, USA
Departments of Physiology[2] and Medicine[3], Hamamatsu University School of Medicine, Hamamatsu 431-31, Japan

Introduction

In the aortic tree, atherosclerotic lesions are distributed preferentially in the branching and curved areas. In these lesion-prone areas, focal accumulation of lipid deposition has been detected in normal and atherosclerotic aortas by using radio-labeled low density lipoprotein (LDL) or Sudanophilic stain (1,2). These observations suggest the importance of hemodynamic factors (e.g., local wall shear stress) for atherogenesis, including the initiation, localization and progression of atherosclerosis.

Vascular endothelium has the function of regulating macromolecular entry and exit between the blood circulation and the subendothelial tissue. Macromolecular transport across the endothelial layer takes place via transcellular or paracellular pathways (3-5). Transcellular pathway occurs via the endocytotic vesicles involving either receptor-mediated or non-receptor-mediated transfer of macromolecules. Macromolecular transport via the paracellular route takes place thorough the cleft between two adjacent endothelial cells and is controlled by the intercellular tight junction. Although the vesicular transport of macromolecules has been questioned because the apparently free vesicles have been shown to be parts of surface membrane invaginations (6-10), its role may depend on the level of the vessel tree and the conditions of the blood and tissue. The purpose of the present investigation is to study the effect of hemodynamics on the junctional transport of macromolecule in relation to atherogenesis.

Junctional transport and endothelial permeability

Macromolecular transport via intercellular junctions is restricted with respect to their molecular size. Recent time-dependent perfusion study has demonstrated that horseradish peroxidase (HRP) can reach the subendothelial space by passing through junctionless clefts of the rat thoracic aorta and that the HRP concentration profile in the junctionless clefts shows a gradient decreasing from the luminal to the abluminal front (10).

Key words: atherosclerosis, endothelium, permeability, shear stress, tight junction.

F-actin, which forms the microfilament network of the cytoskeleton, plays an important structural and mechanical role in maintaining the integrity of individual cells and cell monolayers (11,12). Relocalization and remodeling of actin filaments in the endothelial cell have been shown to be related to the changes in morphology and permeability of the endothelial cell (13). Phallacidin is a mushroom toxin which stabilizes existing actin filaments and enhances polymerization of actin filaments. Pretreatment of phallacidin prevented the changes in actin filament distribution and markedly attenuated the increase in albumin permeability induced by the challenge of inflammatory mediators, including thrombin, in cultured endothelial cells. These data support the hypothesis that actin filaments, particularly the peripheral bands, is a critical factor in the maintenance of the barrier function of endothelial cells (14).

Hemodynamics and the control of endothelial permeability

According to experimental studies performed in our laboratory (15,16) and the recently proposed time-dependent theoretical models (17), changes in transendothelial permeability occur in a narrow window of the endothelial cell cycle such as mitosis and cell death. These studies showed that the widening of intercellular junctions during endothelial cell mitosis leads to the initial entry of macromolecules such as Evans blue labeled albumin (EBA) and LDL into the intima. The detailed relationship between the topographical distributions of mitotic cells and macromolecular leakage, as well as the roles of hemodynamic factors in such distributions and in the preferential localization of atherosclerosis, however, require further analysis.

In the present study, we made detailed mapping of the morphometric parameters of endothelial cells in the rabbit aorta to reveal the local shear patterns. Regions of secondary flow are associated with low shear stress, rounder cell shape, and increased macromolecular leakage. On the other hand, the endothelial cells in high shear regions are elongated and well aligned with the flow direction, and macromolecular permeability is low. The regions of the arterial tree with secondary flow are associated with increase in cell turnover and the opening of tight junctions, which in turn cause an increase in macromolecules transfer from the luminal side to the abluminal side of the endothelial layer (Figure 1).

The peripheral bands and the actin stress fibers of the endothelial cells are increased under high shear condition (18). The regulation of junctional transport by shear stress may be linked to the degree of F-actin rearrangement.

Possible mechanisms for sensing shear force in the endothelium

In the cultured endothelial cells, the effect of shear stress on the endothelial cell has been explored. The flow chamber has been employed to study the effect of shear stresses on gene expression of the endothelial cell.. Tissue plasminogen activator is increased by shear, whereas plasminogen activator inhibitor-1 level is not altered by elevation of shear stress (19).

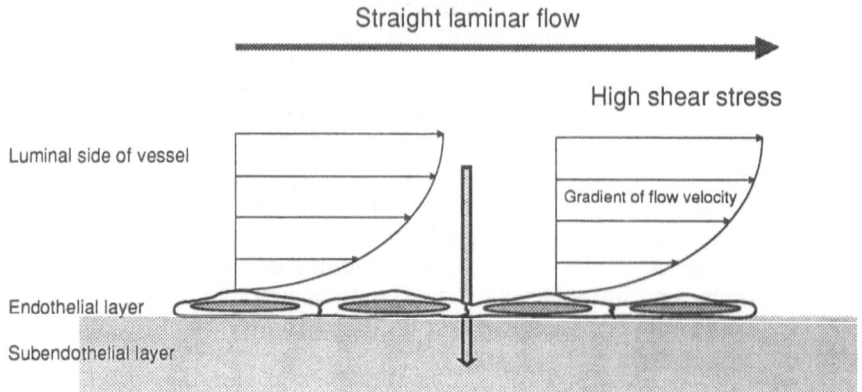

Straight laminar flow

High shear stress

Luminal side of vessel

Gradient of flow velocity

Endothelial layer

Subendothelial layer

Retricted macromolecular transport

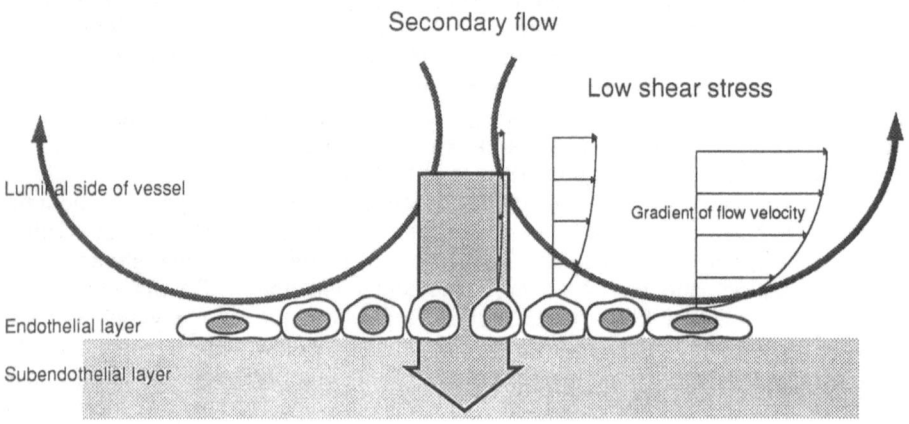

Secondary flow

Low shear stress

Luminal side of vessel

Gradient of flow velocity

Endothelial layer

Subendothelial layer

Increased macromolecular transport

Figure 1   Relationship among flow pattern, shear stress, endothelial cell shape, intercellular junction, and macromolecular permeability.

Under straight laminar flow,   endothelial cells are exposed to shear stresses with mostly uniform direction and high magnitude.   Secondary flows result in random direction and spatially and temporally varying magnitude (which is always less than that observed under straight laminar flow) of shear stresses on the endothelial cells.   This condition may lead to an enhanced endothelial cell turnover,   a reduced integrity of intercellular junctions, and an increase in macromolecular leakage.

stresses on the endothelial cells. This condition may lead to an enhanced endothelial cell turnover, a reduced integrity of intercellular junctions, and an increase in macromolecular leakage.

The mechanism by which hemodynamic forces, such as shear stress, are sensed by the endothelial cell and transduced to intracellular signals, however, are not yet clearly understood. There are unusually high amounts of sialic acids on the surface of the vascular endothelia (20). Pohl has proposed an hypothesis that shear stress acts on structures anchored in the endothelial cell membrane and mechanically enhances the interaction between regulatory proteins and their targets (21). They showed the inhibitory effect of neuraminidase, which removes sialic acids, on the flow-dependent dilation and concluded that sialic acid on the endothelial surface is an integral component of membrane-anchored glycoproteins and lipoproteins, which may act as "mechanoreceptors".

Conclusion

Hemodynamic factors may modulate the cytoskeletal network which affects the endothelial morphology and cell turnover, thus causing the increased macromolecular transport via the paracellular, transjunctional pathway. These changes may provide a mechanism by which hemodynamic factors play an important role in atherogenesis.

References

1. Stemerman M.B., Morrel E.M., Burke K.R., Colton C.K., Smith K.A., and Lees R.S. Local variation in arterial wall permeability to low density lipoprotein in normal rabbit aorta. Arteriosclerosis 1986;6:64-69.
2. Schwenke D.C., and Carew T.E. Initiation of atherosclerotic lesions in cholesterol-fed rabbits.I.Focal increases in arterial LDL concentration precede development of fatty streak lesions. Arteriosclerosis 1989;9:895-907.
3. Malik A.B., Lynch J.J., and Cooper J.A. Endothelial barrier function. J. Invest. Dermatol. 1989;93:62S-67S.
4. Simionescu M. Receptor-mediated transcytosis of plasma molecules by vascular endothelium. In:Simionescu N.,Simionescu M.,editors. Endothelial cell biology in health and disease, New York; Plenum Press. 1988:69-104.
5. Shasby D.M. Endothelial albumin transport in vitro. In:Ryan U.,editor.Endothelial cells. 1988:39-54.
6. Bundgaard M., Frøkjaer-Jensen J., and Crone C. Endothelial plasmalemmal vesicules as elements in a system of branching invaginations from the cell surface. Proc. Natl. Acad. Sci. USA 1979;76:6439-6442.
7. Bundgaard M., Hagman P., and Crone C. The three-dimentional organization of plasmalemmal vesicular profiles in the endothelium of rat heart capillaries. Microvasc. Res. 1983;25:358-68.

9. Frøkjaer-Jensen J.   Three-dimentional organization of plasmalemmal vesicles in endothelial cells. An analysis by serial sectioning of frog mesenteric capillaries.   J. Ultrastruct. Res.   1980;73:9-20.

10. Huang A-L, Jan K-M, and Chien S.   Role of Intercellular Junctions in the Passage of Horseradish Peroxidase Across Aortic Endothelium.   Lab. Invest. 1992;67(2):201-209.

11. Stossel T.P.   Contribution of actin to the structure of the cytoplasmic matrix.   J. Cell. Biol.   1984;99,Suppl.2:15s-21s.

12. Wong M.K.K., and Gotlieb A.I.   Endothelial cell monolayer integrity.I. Characterization of dense peripheral band of microfilaments. Arteriosclerosis   1986;6:212-219.

13. Phillips P. G., and Tsan M-F.   Hypoxia causes increased albumin permeability of cultured endothelial monolayers.   J. Appl. Physiol. 1988;64:1196-1202.

14. Phillips P.G., Lum H., Malik A.B., and Tsan M-F.   Phallacidin prevents thrombin-induced increases in endothelial permeability to albumin.   Am. J. Physiol.   1989;257(26):C562-C567.

15. Lin S-J, Jan K-M, Schuessler G., Weinbaum S., and Chien S.   Enhanced macromolecular permeability of aortic endothelial cells in association with mitosis.   Atherosclerosis   1988;73:223-232.

16. Lin S-J, J an K-M, Weinbaum S., and Chien S.   Transendothelial transport of low density lipoprotein in association with cell mitosis in rat aorta Arteriosclerosis   989;73:230-236.

17. Weinbaum S., Tazeghai G., Ganatos P., Pfeffer R., and Chien S.   Effect of cell turnover and leaky junctions on arterial macromolecular transport.   Am. J. Physiol.   1985;248:H945-H960.

18. Sato M., Levesque M.J., and Nerm R.M.   Micropipette aspiration of cultured bovine aortic endothelial cells exposed to shear stress.   Arteriosclerosis 1987;7:276-286.

19. Diamond S.L., Eskin S.G., and McIntire L.V.   Fluid flow stimulates tissue plasminogen activator secretion by cultured human endothelial cells. Science   1989;243:1483-1485.

20. Born G.V.R., and Palinski W.   Unusually high concentrations of sialic acids on the surface of vascular endothelia.   Br. J. Exp. Pathol.   1985;66:543-549.

21. Pohl U., Herlan K., Huang A., and Bassenge E.   EDRF-mediated shear-induced dilation opposes myogenic vasoconstriction in small rabbit arteries.   Am. J. Physiol.   1991;261(30):H2016-H2023.

Fibrinolysis

THE PHYSIOLOGY OF THE FIBRINOLYTIC SYSTEM

AKIKAZU TAKADA   Department of Physiology, Hamamatsu University
School of Medicine, Hamamatsu-shi,, Shizuoka-ken, Japan 431-31

INTRODUCTION

There are many publications on the biochemical aspects of fibrinolysis
and therapeutic effects of thrombolytic drugs in occlusive vessel
diseases such as myocardial infarction, cerebrovascular thrombosis and
venous thrombosis predisposing to pulmonary embolism.   Fibrinolysis
is, however, physiological phenomenon, which is constantly operating
together with the coagulation system to secure the sufficient blood
flow to peripheral organs or tissues.   We have examined effects of
various physiological parameters on the fibrinolytic enzyme system,
which will be reviewed together with results reported from other
laboratories.

AGE

It is well known that the incidence of thrombotic diseases increase in
older age.   Fibrinolytic activity appears to be present in the blood
early in fetal life.   Plasminogen has been detected in the blood of
10.5 week embryo, levels rising through fetal life.   Plasminogen
concentration is, however, low in the newborn, usually around 50 % of
adult values, and reaches the adult levels rapidly.   There are also
many reports suggesting increases in various coagulation factors in the
aged.   We have measured t-PA antigen, PA activity and PA inhibitor
activity in various age groups.   Antigen levels of t-PA increased with
age.   Since t-PA exists not only in the free form but in the complex
with various inhibitors such as PAI-1 or α_2AP, there is a possibility
that an increase in t-PA antigen is due to an increase in t-PA-PAI-1
complex, thus active t-PA levels decreasing.   We then measured
plasma levels of PA inhibitor activity and PA activity, the latter
representing the concentration of free t-PA levels.   PA inhibitor
activity increased and PA activity decreased with age, which correlates
well with the higher incidence of thrombotic disease in the aged.
Plasma plasminogen levels did not change between 2 years old to 90
years old.

SEX

It has been repeatedly shown that the incidence of thrombotic disease
is less in females than in males.   A possible explanation lies in the
different endocrine make-up of men and women.   In fact, the
cardiovascular disease incidence was lower in premenopausal than
postmenopausal women.   We have shown that plasma levels of t-PA
antigen were higher in males than females, and those in females
gradually increased with increase in age, reaching the same levels as
those of males at their 60s.   Plasma levels of t-PA-PAI-1 complex were
also higher in males than females, indicating that t-PA was mainly in
the form of a complex with PAI-1 in males.   Plasma levels of free PAI-

117

1 were higher in males than in females up to their 60s, suggesting that male blood was less fibrinolytic than female blood. In fact euglobulin clot lysis time was faster in females than in males.

CIRCADIAN FLUCTUATION

There is a circadian variation in the incidence of stroke, myocardial infarction and sudden death. The analysis of data revealed the high incidence of onset of pain of myocardial infarction between 6 am and 12 noon. The higher vascular tone in the morning was implicated in the high incidence of myocardial infarction. The possibility exists, however, that there is high coagulability and low fibrinolytic activity in the morning. Fearnly and his coworkers first noted the circadian variation of fibrinolytic activity, showing that fibrinolysis was considerably higher in the afternoon. Since then many groups of workers have confirmed the results. Analysis of the blood fibrinolytic components indicated that t-PA activity increased from 9 am to 3 pm, and that both t-PA and PAI-1 antigen levels decreased in the afternoon. We have shown that euglobulin clot lysis time (ELT) was longer in the morning and gradually shortened in the afternoon in both males and females, ELT of females being shorter than that of males. Plasma levels of t-PA, free PAI-1 and t-PA-PAI-1 complex were high in the morning, decreasing towards evening. Those values were lower in females than in males. Similar circadian variation of fibrinolytic parameters was recognized in patients with angina pectoris. It is now clear that higher fibrinolytic activity in the afternoon is mainly due to the decreased release of PAI-1 from endothelial cells, not due to increase in t-PA release.
Higher coagulability in the morning may also be related to the higher activity of platelet. Serotonin contents of platelets are higher in the morning and decrease in the afternoon. Serotonin released from platelets causes the contraction of smooth muscle of blood vessel.

ALCOHOL, SMOKING AND MENTAL STRESS

There has been strong interest among epidemiologists in the relationships between risk factors and atherosclerosis and occlusive cardiovascular disease. As to effects of alcohol ingestion on fibrinolysis, some investigators reported hyperfibrinolysis, and the other observed decreased plasma fibrinolytic activity. Several epidemiologic studies have demonstrated a negative correlation between alcohol consumption and fatal ischemic heart disease. This preventive role of ethanol has been attributed to increase in the concentration of high-density lipoprotein (HDL) in the plasma as well as to the decreased aggregability of platelets. We have examined the acute effects of alcohol ingestion in plasma fibrinolytic activity and platelet serotonin metabolism. Ingestion of 250 ml of whisky (43 % of alcohol v/v) did not result in any change in fibrinolytic parameters such as t-PA or PAI-1 in the plasma compared with controls who took tea. Euglobulin clot lysis time prolonged on the next morning due not to decrease in the release of t-PA but to the increase in the release of PAI-1. On the other hand, platelet activity including serotonin uptake was inhibited immediately after alcohol ingestion. One half of alcohol's protection action against coronary heart disease appears to be caused not by hyperfibrinolysis but increased HDL levels, and the rest will be mediated by significant alcohol-induced inhibition of platelet function as its aggregation, adhesion and thromboxane A2 release.
In comparing groups of heavy smokers, many investigators reported on decrease in fibrinolysis There were no reports on the effects of short-term smoking, although no change in plasma fibrinogen has been

noted following one cigarette smoking. Our results on the effects of short-term smoking indicated that both PA and PAI-activities increased after cigarette smoking. Especially plasma t-PA antigen levels increased after smoking. Plasma epinephrine levels also increased, which may be related to the increased release of t-PA after cigarette smoking.

Physical and mental stress were reported to influence the activity of coagulation. Macfarlane and Biggs noted that nearly 50 % of patients showed increase in fibrinolytic activity when given premedication prior to an operation. The fear of the impending operation was considered to be the major factor in influencing fibrinolysis. The impending venopuncture and medical examination were used to test fibrinolysis, confirming that fear was the factor to cause enhanced fibrinolysis, possibly through changed in sympathetic nervous activity. We took advantage of the bleeding time test in which students cut the ear of their colleagues and measured time for the cessation of bleeding. The procedure was fearful because students did not know the extent of pain incurred by the incision, and the precision of the technique used by their non-skilled friends. We intentionally stressed the fact that the incision must be large enough to secure the reasonable extent of bleeding. The results indicate that students showed dramatic increase in fibrinolysis as measured by shortening of ELT even after the verbal explanation of the procedure. The test of the bleeding time itself also shortened ELT, but to less extent compared with the effects of verbal explanation. The analysis of changes in fibrinolytic parameters revealed decrease in the release of PAI-1 from endothelial cells. When platelet responses were analyzed, increase in the response to serotonin, and ADP was noted. Plasma levels of serotonin, epinephrine and norepinephrine increased after bleeding time procedure. It is possible that mental stress enhanced fibrinolytic activity by lowering plasma levels of PAI-1, which may be caused by changes in sympathetic nerve activity.

EXERCISE

Since Biggs et al reported on enhanced fibrinolysis upon exercise, many groups demonstrated increase in blood fibrinolysis using a wide variety of exercise forms Increase in fibrinolysis was shown to be due to a rise in plasminogen activator level, which may be caused by adrenergic stimulation. If changes in plasminogen activator, pulse rate and catecholamine level are examined at intervals after exercise, plasminogen activator and pulse rate rise in parallel with increase in workload, whereas catecholamines increase only after exhaustive exercise. Furthermore, when b-blockers are used at the time of catecholamine infusion, plasminogen activator response can only be partially blocked. The similar results have been observed in exercise, thus it is now suggested that fibrinolysis induced by exercise is not mediated via b-adrenergic receptors. Except for changes in plasminogen activator after exercise, little changes have been reported in plasma levels of fibrinogen and plasminogen. Antiplasmin levels hardly change. As to plasma levels of fibrinogen degradation products (FDP), there is still controversy. Some workers have been unable to show any change in serum FDP concentration, but others have shown two to four fold increase.

We have examined changes in fibrinolytic parameters with myocardial infarction. Plasma levels of t-PA increased and PAI-1 decreased after exercise in normal persons. Basic levels of PAI-1 were higher in patients with myocardial infarction. In fact one of our patients showed a high level of PAI-1 just before the onset of myocardial infarction. When comparison was made between patients with single vs multivessel disease, PAI-1 levels were high in patients with multivessel disease. The extent of increase in t-PA after exercise was less in patients with multivessel disease. PAI activity as well as plasma levels of PAI-1 decreased more after exercise in patients with multivessel disease, which may mean that exercise is of protective value in patients with myocardial infarction.

EMOTION AND ITS DISORDERS

Some lines of evidence suggest that disturbances in the regulation of circadian rhythms may be of prime importance in the pathophysiology of depression. It has been also reported that patients with affective disorders have a higher than expected rate of mortality from cardiovascular disease. Further evidence suggests that major depression has a direct negative impact on the outcome of cardiovascular disease. We have measured change in fibrinolytic parameters in patients with neurosis or depression. Patients with depression and neurosis had lower levels of t-PA in plasma. Neurotic patients seemed to have lower levels of t-PA than depressive patients. Plasma levels of free PAI-1 and t-PA-PAI-1 complex were lower in depression and neurotic patients than in normal controls. ELT was shorter in depressive and neurotic patients, mainly due to the lower release of PAI-1 from endothelial cells.

NUTRITION AND BODY WEIGHT

In general, many data suggest that lipaemia inhibits fibrinolysis. However, the mechanism of fat-induced inhibition is not elucidated. In lipaemia, there is chylomicron in plasma, which is known to have antifibrinolytic activity in vitro and in vivo. Beta-lipoprotein, which rises after fat ingestion, also has antifibrinolytic activity. It is shown that increase in plasma levels of triglyceride results in increase in plasma levels of PAI-1 concentration. In the case of high triglyceride levels, VLDL of larger particle sizes caused the release of PAI-1 from cultured endothelial cells. We have had volunteers take butter (50 or 100 grams) at 8:30 and measured fibrinolytic parameters and platelet aggregability. It was shown that ELT of volunteers loaded with 100 g of butter significantly prolonged at 14:30 and 16:30 compared with controls or 50 g butter loaded volunteers. PAI-1 also significantly increased at 10:30, two hours after fat intake, which means that triglyceride induced the release of PAI-1. Platelet response to ADP and collagen was inhibited. These results suggest that lipaemia itself is thrombogenic with respect to fibrinolysis, but antithrombogenic in platelet activity. Probably, the prolonged presence of lipaemia results in atherosclerosis, which causes thrombosis.
There is a general agreement on decrease in fibrinolytic activity in obesity. There was an inverse relationship between body weight and fibrinolytic activity in normal persons. The reduction of fibrinolysis in obese people seems to be mainly due to decrease in plasma levels of t-PA. Fibrinolysis was not only reduced in a resting condition, but the response to exercise or venous occlusion was also impaired in obesity.
We measured various fibrinolytic parameters in normal controls and diabetic patients. Body weight positively correlated with t-PA, PAI-1 and ELT in normal subjects. The prolongation of ELT is considered to be caused by increase in plasma levels of PAI-1. It is indicated that PAI-1 was correlated with insulin levels in both normal subjects and diabetic patients. Apparent correlations between PAI-1 and body weight or triglyceride levels may reflect the fact that insulin levels were correlated with both body weight and triglyceride levels. In diabetic patients, correlations between body weight and fibrinolytic parameters were obscure in contrast to good correlations in normal subjects. It is

suggested that the regulatory mechanisms which underlie the relation of body weight to fibrinolytic parameters are impaired in diabetes mellitus.

ROLES OF FIBRINOLYSIS IN CELL GROWTH AND MIGRATION

It was shown that activated macrophages and transformed tumor cells produced u-PA. Since then numerous reports have been published concerning the roles of plasminogen activator in cell growth and migration, especially metastasis of tumor cells. The presence of u-PA, PAI-1 and PAI-2 in tumor cells has been shown by the quantitative determination of these factors and immunohistochemical stainings. We have shown increases in u-PA, PAI-1 and PAI-2, but no change or rather a decrease in t-PA in tumor tissue in stomach cancer, ovarian and uterine tumor, breast cancer, and colon cancer.

If roles of u-PA are to activate plasminogen, the inhibition of u-PA by PAI-1 should result in the inhibition of proliferation and metastasis of tumors. The concentrations of u-PA and PAI-1 in tumor tissues are higher in proportion to the tumor size, and tumors with metastasis have large amounts of u-PA and PAI-1. On the other hand, tumors with high levels of PAI-2 stay in smaller sizes and are less metastatic. These results may indicate that roles of PAI-1 and PAI-2 in tumor growth and metastasis are different, PAI-1 being facilitative, and PAI-2 being inhibitory. There are various hypotheses to explain differences of functions of PAI-1 and PAI-2, but further studies are definitely needed.

PREGNANCY AND PUERPERIUM

There is a general consensus that fibrinolysis decreases during pregnancy. The decrease starts at about twelfth week of pregnancy and continues up to around 26th week, thus reaching a plateau. ELT prolongs at these periods. It is claimed that plasma levels of PAI-1 remain constant, and that there are marked increases in the levels of $a_2$macroglobulin and $a_2$antiplasmin. Because of the diminished response to venous occlusion, it is suggested that impairment of the synthesis and release of t-PA may be the major cause of the decrease of fibrinolysis during pregnancy. During labor, in spite of strenuous physical activity and mental stress, fibrinolytic activity remains low, however fibrinolysis abruptly increases after delivery. Such rise takes places before the umbilical cord is clamped and while the placenta is still in situ. Placental separation seems to be much responsible, however, for the further rise in fibrinolysis at parturition. We have measured plasma levels of t-PA and u-PA in pregnant women, and found either t-PA or u-PA levels did not increase significantly in the first and second trimesters, but both activators increased after the third trimester of pregnancy. The high levels of PAs continued throughout the first stage of labor. The levels of t-PA further increased for the first few hours after delivery, whereas the levels of u-PA returned to normal immediately following childbirth. In order to know the roles of the uterus or placenta in the elevated levels of PAs, we took samples from the uterine venous blood. There was no significant difference in the levels of t-PA antigens in between peripheral and venous blood in the third trimester of pregnancy. The levels of t-PA were higher, however, after than before delivery. The results indicate that the uterus is involved in the high levels of t-PA in the circulation. Further increase in t-PA in the post partum may be explained by the possibility that the involuting uterus produces large amounts of t-PA. As stated above the separation of the placenta may partly be responsible for the high levels of t-PA in the

circulation due to the damage to the endothelium in the placental bed.
Plasminogen activators are implicated also in the ovulation. Roles of
plasminogen activator in the follicle rupture has been proposed, based
upon the observations that plasmin is capable of weakening follicle
wall strips in vitro, and that increasing amounts of plasminogen
activators are produced by rat granulosa cells toward the time of
ovulation. We have induced the ovulation in rat by the injection of
human chorionic gonadotropin (HCG), and measured the concentration of
PA in the ovarian extract.   The concentration of PA dramatically
increased up to just before the ovulation and then dropped to low
levels after the ovulation. These processes were shown to be
independent of prostaglandin systems . These results also raise the
possibility that PA is involved for the degradation of the supporting
structure such as collagen or elastin, and leading to the rupture of
ovarian follicles.

FIBRINOLYSIS IN PHYSIOLOGY

Fibrinolytic system has evolved to remove fibrin clots formed at
injury, and to facilitate blood flow to secure recanalization of a
blood vessel. Blood clots are not only formed at the site of vascular
injury, but on the atheromatous plaques, leading to thrombosis.
Physiological stimuli to control the synthesis and release of t-PA and
PAI-1 are still far from clear. Renewed efforts to clarify the
physiological regulation of fibrinolysis are expected in the future.
We cite here mainly our review and books in this field as references .
The review of the physiology of fibrinolytic system will be published
in Japanese Journal of Physiology in this fall.

REFERENCES

1. Marsh N (1981) Fibrinolysis. John Wiley & Sons, Chichester

2. Ogston D (1983) The physiology of hemostasis. Croom Helm, London.

3. Castellino FJ, Gaffney PJ, Samama MM and Takada A (1986)
   Fundamental and clinical fibrinolysis. Elsevier Science Publishers
   BV, Amsterdam.

4. Takada A and Takada Y (1988) Physiology of plasminogen. Haemostasis
   18(suppl. 1).: 25-35

5. Takada A, Samama MM and Collen D (1990) Protease inhibitors.
   Elsevier Science Publishers, Amsterdam

6. Schmitt M, Jänicke F and Graeff H (1992) Fibrinolysis 6(suppl 4)

7.Takada A and Buzynski AZ (1992) Hemostasis and circulation.
   Springer-Verlag, Tokyo.

8 Takada A and Takada Y (1992) The physiology of the fibrinolytic
   system. Jap J Physiol 42: in press

CONFORMATIONAL CHANGE OF GLU-PLASMINOGEN: EFFECTS OF N-TERMINAL PEPTIDES OF GLU-PLASMINOGEN

YUMIKO TAKADA, TETSUMEI URANO, SATOMI TAKAHASHI, KENJI SAKAKIBARA AND AKIKAZU TAKADA Department of Physiology, Hamamatsu University, School of Medicine, Hamamatsu, Shizuoka, 431-31, Japan

INTRODUCTION

Native plasminogen with glutamic acid at the N-terminus (Glu-plg) has a tight conformation possibly due to the binding of the N-terminal part to the lysine binding sites (LBS) on kringle 1 (1, 2) or kringle 4 (3) or kringle 5 through amino-hexyl (AH) site (4). Lysine analogues, therefore, could alter the conformation of Glu-plg to looser form (5, 6, 7) by dissociating the N-terminal peptides from LBS or AH site. Fig. 1 shows the schematic explanation of the conformation of Glu-plg and Lys-plg.

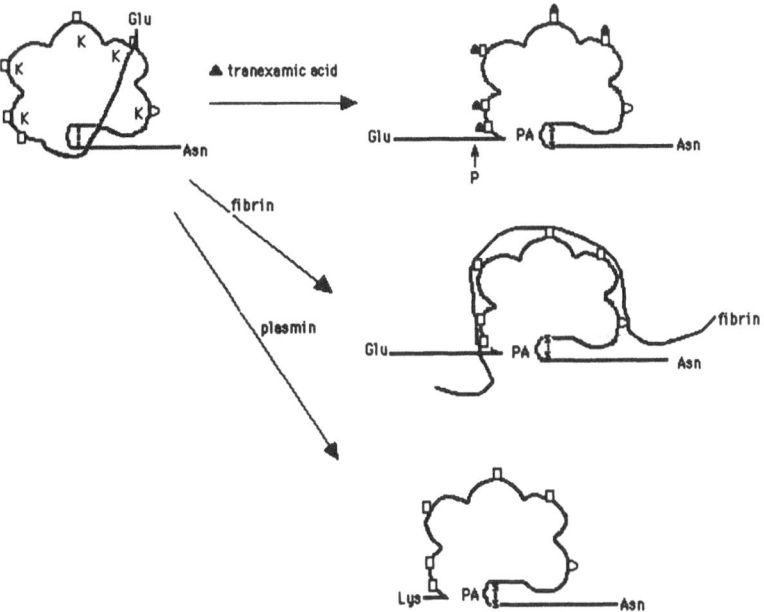

Fig. 1 Scheme of conformation of Glu-plg and Lys-plg
"Glu" or "Lys" : N-terminal aminoacid of Glu-plg. "Asn" : C-terminal aminoacid of Glu-plg. "K": kringle. "P": plasmin. "PA": activator Glu-plg has a tight conformation, because N-terminal portion of Glu-plg binds with LBS of kringle 4. Tranexamic acid (lysine analogue) or fibrin alters the conformation of Glu-plg to the looser form. Lys-plg has a looser form, since it is generated by the cleavage of $Lys^{76}-Lys^{77}$ peptide bond of Glu-plg by plasmin.

In order to bind to LBS, lysine analogues such as EACA (epsilon aminocaproic acid) or tranexamic acid must have positively charged amino group at N-terminus and negatively charged carboxyl group at the distance close to these groups of lysine. There is only one peptide sequence where a positively charged group (lysine) is located next to a negatively charged carboxyl group contributed by glutamic acid, that is Lys[50], and Wiman and Wallen reported that Ala[44]-Lys[50] of Glu-plg could be a candidate for N-terminal region for this binding to keep a tight conformation (8). We synthesized Ala[44]-Ser[49] (A-S), Ala[44]-Lys[50] (A-K) and Ala[44]-Glu[51] (A-E), and showed that Ala[44]-Lys[50] and Ala[44]-Glu[51] enhanced the activation of Glu-plg by urokinase (UK) and the conversion of Glu-plg to Lys-plg (9). In this report we showed the enhancement of the activation of plasminogen by tissue plasminogen activator (t-PA) by these peptides. Then the effects on fibrinolysis by these peptides were investigated by euglobulin and fibrin clot lysis times (ECLT and FCLT). To test other lysine residue of N terminal region of Glu-plg, four peptides, Val[17]-Gly[23] (V-G), Lys[19]-Gly[23] (K-G), Lys[19]-Gln[21] (K-Q), Lys[19]-Lys[20] (K-K), were synthesized, and we investigated their effects on the activation of plasminogen by activators and the effects on fibrinolysis.

EFFECTS OF N-TERMINAL PEPTIDES ON THE ACTIVATION OF GLU-PLG BY ACTIVATORS

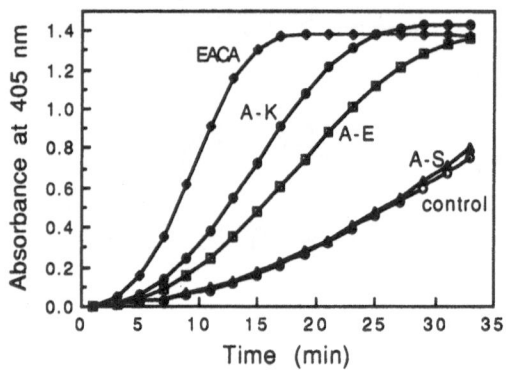

Fig. 2

Effects of peptides on the activation of Glu-plg by tct-PA

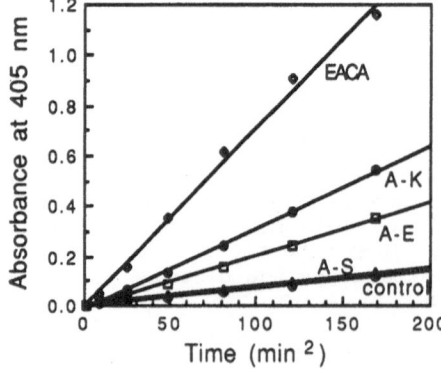

Fig. 3

Activation rate of Glu-plg by tct-PA in the presence of peptides

The assays were performed using a microtiter plate at 37°C in buffer containing 50 mM Tris-HCl with 100 mM NaCl, pH 7.4. Glu-plg or Lys-plg (0.5 μM) was activated by two-chain tissue plasminogen activator (tct-PA: 200 nM for Glu-plg, 5 nM for Lys-plg) in the presence or absence of N-terminal peptide (2 mM) and the hydrolysis of S-2251 (0.3 mM) was monitored at 405 nm by automatic microtiter plate reader. Fig. 2 shows the effects of peptides near Lys[50] (A-S, A-K and A-E) on the activation of Glu-plg by tct-PA. Epsilon aminocaproic acid (EACA) was used as a lysine analogue which enhances the activation of Glu-plg by activators. Activation rate of Glu-plg was determined by using the slope of plot of A_{405} vs t^2 (Fig. 3). From Fig. 3 activation rate of Glu-plg by tct-PA was calculated as 0.69×10^{-3} A_{405}/min^2, and that in the presence of A-K, A-E, A-S or EACA was 3.27×10^{-3}, 2.11×10^{-3}, 0.74×10^{-3} and 7.15×10^{-3} A_{405}/min^2, respectively. These results indicated that A-K, A-E and EACA enhanced the activation of Glu-plg by tct-PA. Effects of other four peptides near Lys[19] (V-G, K-G, K-Q, K-K) on the activation of Glu-plg by tct-PA were also measured. Only K-K had an enhancing effect. No peptides enhanced the activation of Lys-plg by tct-PA. We have reported that the enhancement of the activation by A-K and A-E was observed when urinary plasminogen activator (u-PA) was used as an activator.(9). This time we determined the effects of four peptides near Lys[19] (V-G, K-G, K-Q, K-K) on the activation of Glu-plg by u-PA. K-K also enhanced the activation of Glu-plg by u-PA. Results were summarized in Table 1.

Table 1

Effects of peptides on the activation of Glu-plg by activators

	A-K	A-E	A-S	K-K	EACA
Glu-plg + t-PA	507.4	310.3	104.3	345.3	1036.2
Lys-plg + t-PA	92.0	98.1	99.5	95.6	96.0
Glu-plg + u-PA	493.5	235.8	97.8	186.1	521.7
Lys-plg + u-PA	64.2	84.5	87.6	90.2	71.1

Each number represents the mean of 3 points. Numbers are shown as %. The activity of the mixture of plasminogen and activator in the absence of peptides was designated as 100 %. Results in the presence of V-G, K-G and K-Q were not shown, since these peptides did not have any effects on the activation of plasminogen by activators.

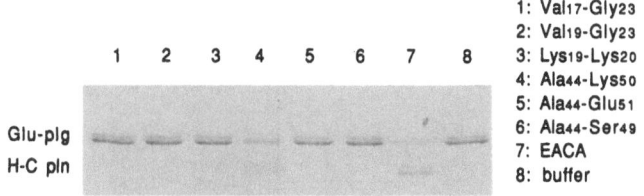

1: Val17-Gly23
2: Val19-Gly23
3: Lys19-Lys20
4: Ala44-Lys50
5: Ala44-Glu51
6: Ala44-Ser49
7: EACA
8: buffer

Fig. 4 Activation of Glu-plg by tct-PA in the presence of peptides "H-C pln" indicates the heavy chain of plasmin.

SDS-PAGE was used to show the enhanced plasmin formation from Glu-plg activated by tct-PA (Fig. 4). Glu-plg (2 μM) was incubated with tct-PA (200 nM), aprotinin (10 u/ml) with various peptides (1.6 mM) at 37°C for 30 min. The conversion from Glu-plg to plasmin was examined by the reduced SDS-PAGE. In Fig. 4 it is shown that EACA and A-K significantly enhanced the conversion from Glu-plg to plasmin, and K-K slightly enhanced it.

EFFECTS OF N-TERMINAL PEPTIDES ON ACTIVATORS

Effects of N-terminal peptides on the activity of u-PA were measured using the hydrolysis of S-2444 by u-PA. The hydrolysis of S-2444 (0.2 mM) by u-PA (5 nM) were measured in the presence of various N-terminal peptides (2 mM). No peptides had enhancing nor inhibiting effect on the activity of u-PA. Activity of tct-PA (50 nM) in the presence of various N-terminal peptides (2 mM) were measured by the hydrolysis of S-2288 (0.2 mM). No effects were observed on the activity of t-PA in the presence of peptides.

EFFECTS OF N-TERMINAL PEPTIDE ON FIBRINOLYSIS

We used euglobulin clot lysis time (ECLT) for measuring fibrinolysis. Euglobulin clot was made by mixing with tct-PA (2.5 nM) or u-PA (5 nM) and thrombin (25 u/ml) in the presence of peptide in the microtiter plate at 37°C, and the turbidity of clot was measured every 5 min by the microtiter plate reader with 340 nm of wavelength.

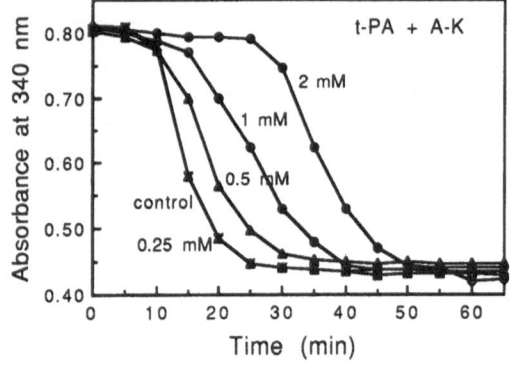

Fig. 5

Euglobulin clot lysis time by t-PA in the presence of various concentrations of A-K

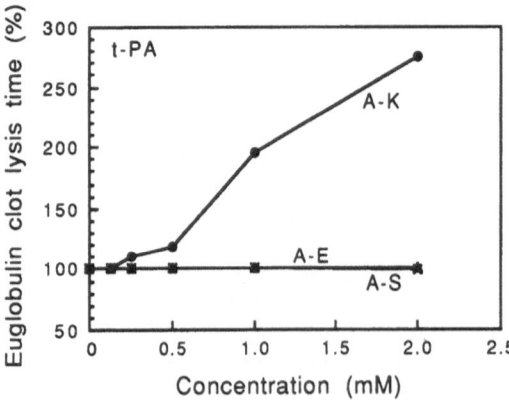

Fig. 6

Effects of various concentrations of A-K, A-E and A-S on ECLT activated by tct-PA

High absorbance (OD_{340Max}) represents the turbidity of the euglobulin clot. When euglobulin clot was dissolved totally, constant lower absorbance was obtained (OD_{340Min}). The point of half lysis was determined as ECLT, which was obtained by the calculation as midpoint between OD_{340Max} and OD_{340Min}. ECLT was also done in purified system. We measured fibrin clot lysis time (FCLT) of the mixture of Glu-plg (0.2 μM) or Lys-plg (0.2 μM), tct-PA (3 nM) or u-PA (2.4 nM), thrombin (20 u/ml), fibrinogen (8 μM) and peptide (2 mM).

The patterns of euglobulin clot lysis were shown in Fig. 5. Fig. 5 shows the effects of various concentration of A-K on euglobulin clot lysis by tct-PA. From this figure ECLT was calculated. ECLT without peptide was 14 min. ECLT were calculated as 14 min, 18 min, 25 min and 35 min in the presence of 0.25 mM, 0.5 mM, 1 mM and 2 mM A-K, respectively. These results show that euglobulin clot lysis was inhibited by A-K.

Inhibitory activities were calculated as "(ECLT with peptide/ECLT without peptide) x 100". Fig. 6 shows the inhibitory effects of various concentrations of A-K, A-E and A-S on ECLT activated by tct-PA. A-K has dose dependent inhibitory effect on ECLT activated by tct-PA, but A-E and A-S did not have inhibitory effects. Effects of various concentrations of these three peptide on ECLT activated by u-PA were also investigated. Results were same as those by tct-PA. That is, A-K dose dependently inhibited the ECLT activated by u-PA.

Effects of various peptides (2 mM) on ECLT were summarized in Table 2. 2 mM of EACA completely inhibited ECLT and FCLT.

Table 2

Effects of peptides on ECLT

	A-K	A-E	A-S	V-G	K-G	K-Q	K-K
ECLT-u-PA	204	115	114	100	106	98	147
Glu-plg-u-PA	126	112	119	112	108	112	145
Lys-plg-u-PA	144	117	100	114	110	100	100
ECLT-t-PA	276	101	99	98	115	100	121
Glu-plg-t-PA	145	111	103	104	104	100	123
Lys-plg-t-PA	135	100	104	108	115	102	112

Each number represents the mean of 3 points. Numbers are shown as %. ECLT without peptides was designated as 100 %. Concentration of peptides was 2 mM.

DISCUSSION AND SUMMARY

We reported A-K and A-E enhanced the activation of Glu-plg by u-PA in a dose dependent manner similar to EACA, but A-S did not have any effects. These peptides, however, did not have enhancing effects on the activation of Lys-plg by u-PA. A-K and A-E enhanced the conversion of Glu-plg to Lys-plg (9). A-E had less enhancing effects than A-K. One of the reason might be that A-K has NH^{3+} and COO^- groups identical to EACA, but COO^- group provided by Glu[51] of A-E does not have exact distance from N-terminal amino group of Lys[50]. The other reason might be that AH site, which prefers lysine side chain of proteins, is not the binding site. From these experiments we concluded that A-K or A-E binds to LBS of kringle 1 or 4 and alters the tight conformation of Glu-plg to looser form.

In this report we investigated the effects of A-K, A-E and A-S on the activation of Glu-plg or Lys-plg by t-PA, and found that A-K and A-E enhanced the activation of Glu-plg, but not Lys-plg (Figs. 2 and 3). These were the same results when we used u-PA as an activator. Then we synthesized four peptides near Lys^{20}, V-G, K-G, K-Q and K-K, although we do not think other lysine residue of N-terminal peptide may be candidates for binding to LBS of kringles of Glu-plg, since they do not have exact distance between N-terminal amino group of lysine and COO^- provided by C-terminal amino acid, but V-G, K-G and K-Q have lysine in the structure. Only K-K had the enhancing effects on the activation of Glu-plg, but not Lys-plg, by u-PA or t-PA (Table 1) The mechanism of the enhancing effects of K-K may be binding of lysine residue to LBS of plasminogen, because of the similar structure of K-K to EACA, not because of the part of peptides near Lys^{20}.

Effects of these seven peptides on fibrinolysis were determined. A-K and K-K inhibited ECLT. The mechanism of inhibition may be the same as EACA, since EACA completely inhibited fibrinolysis although EACA and A-K or K-K enhanced the activation of Glu-plg by activators. Fibrin can not bind to plasminogen because LBS of kringles were occupied by A-K or K-K like EACA.

In conclusion, these studies suggest that A-E may comprise a responsible binding site in the N-terminal portion of Glu-plg to make its tight conformation, and LBS of kringle 1 or 4 is the binding site of N-terminal portion of Glu-plg.

REFERENCES

1. Wiman B. and Collen D. (1978) Nature 272: 548-549

2. Lerch P.G., Rickli E.E., Lergier W. and Gillessen D. (1980) Eur J Biochem 107: 7-13

3. Cummings H.S. and Castellino F.J. (1985) Arch Biochem Biophys 236: 612-618

4. Christensen U (1984) Biochem J 223: 413-421

5. Violand B.N., Byrne R. and Castellino F.J. (1978) J Biol Chem 253: 5395-5401

6. Takada A, Takada Y. and Sugawara Y. (1984) Thromb Res 33: 461-469

7. Sjöholm I., Wiman B. and Wallen P. Eur J Biochem (1973) 39: 471-479

8. Wiman B. and Wallen P. (1975) Eur J Biochem 50: 489-494

9. Urano T., Takada Y. and Takada A. (1991) Thromb Res 61: 349-359

Effect of Calcium Ion on the Euglobulin Clot Lysis Time: Significant shortening by physiological concentration of calcium ion.

Yumi Kozima, Tetsumei Urano*, Kenji Sakakibara*, Kiyohito Serizawa*, Yumiko Takada* and Akikazu Takada*

Departments of Medicine and Physiology*, Hamamatsu University School of Medicine, Handa-cho, Hamamatsu, 431-31, Japan

INTRODUCTION

Euglobulin clot lysis time (ECLT) assay has been considered to be useful to assess the systemic fibrinolytic activity [1] [2].   ECLT is respected to show mainly the activity of tissue plasminogen activator (tPA), since antibody against tPA significantly prolonged ECLT.   We have recently shown, however, that ECLT is primarily determined by the amounts of plasminogen activator inhibitor type 1 (PAI-1) due to the fact that ECLT inversely correlates with the concentration of PAI-1 whereas it did not have any meaningful correlation with tPA antigen level [3].   Taken together these results suggest that the activity of tPA either in plasma or in the euglobulin fraction is controlled by the balance of the concentrations of tPA and PAI-1 and that ECLT reflects the amounts of the active form of tPA which is not bound to PAI-1.   We also recently showed that the addition of kaolin to ECLT (kaolin activated ECLT), in which the contact phase of both the coagulation and fibrinolysis is fully activated, significantly shortened regular ECLT, suggesting that intrinsic fibrinolytic pathway is not mainly involved in regular ECLT [3].   In this paper we report another pathway to enhance ECLT which is induced by the addition of physiological concentration of calcium ion.   We believe it important because Ca^{2+} has been considered to work only to prolong fibrinolysis.

MATERIALS AND METHODS

Plasma sample
Blood samples were obtained from apparently healthy volunteers.   Platelet poor plasma was prepared by the centrifugation of citrated blood (whole blood was mixed with 0.1 vol. of 3.8% sodium citrate) at approximately 2,000 x g for 10 min. at 4°C.   All the platelet poor plasma was kept at -70°C until use.

Plasma euglobulin fraction
The plasma euglobulin fraction was prepared by 20 times dilution of citrated plasma and acidification at pH 5.2.   After leaving for 1 hour at 4°C followed by the centrifugation at approximately 2,000 x g for 10 min. at 4°C, the precipitate was dissolved by the original volume of 0.1 M Tris-HCl buffer pH 7.4.   All the samples were used for ECLT immediately after preparation.

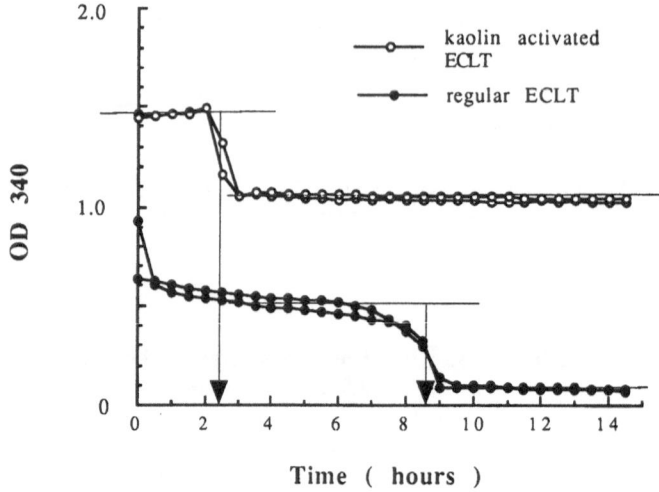

Time (hours)

Fig.1 Regular ECLT and kaolin activated ECLT.
The ordinate shows OD340 and the abscissa shows incubation time.   Euglobulin
clot was made in the microtiter plate in the presence or absence of kaolin, and
the turbidity of the clot was measured every 30 min. by the microtiter plate
reader with 340nm of wave-length.   Arrows show obtained ECLT and kaolin
activated ECLT from the figure.

Euglobulin clot lysis assay (ECLT)
ECLT was assayed by 96-well microtiter plate as previously reported [4-6].   All
the samples were assayed in duplicate.

Kaolin activated ECLT
Kaolin activated ECLT was measured as regular ECLT in the presence of kaolin
suspension (2.5 mg/ml).   The representative data and the procedure to get both
regular ECLT and kaolin activated ECLT are shown in Fig.1.

Proteins
Fibrinogen was obtained from KabiVitrum, Stockholm, Sweden and contaminated
plasminogen was removed by passing through Lysine-sepharose.   Glu-
plasminogen was purified from fresh frozen plasma as previously reported. [7]
t-PA was kindly provided from Sumitomo pharmaceutical company, Osaka, Japan
and human a-thrombin was a kind gift from Green Cross, Osaka, Japan.

Barium-absorbed plasma
All steps were performed at 4°C. $BaCl_2$ was added dropwise (80 ml/liter plasma)
to the plasma and the mixture was stirred for 20 min.   The precipitate was
removed by centrifugation at 10,000 x g for 20 min. at 4°C.   The supernatant
plasma was dialyzed against 0.02M HEPES, 0.15M NaCl, pH 7.4, and was used as
barium-absorbed plasma.

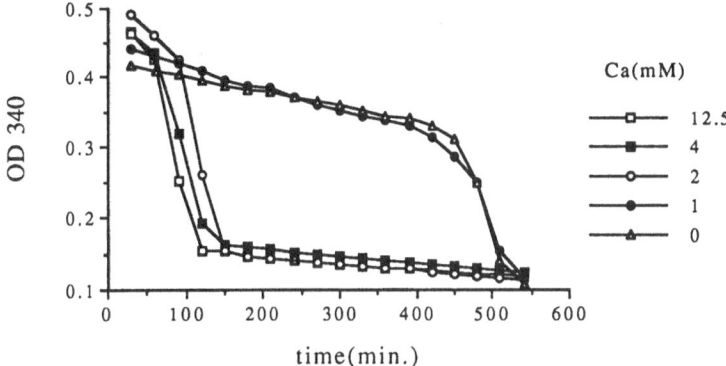

Fig.2 The effect of Ca²⁺ on ECLT
100μl of euglobulin fraction, 25μl of CaCl₂ (final 0, 0.1, 0.5, 1, 2, 4, 8, 12.5mM) and 25μl of 0.1M Tris-HCl buffer pH 7.4 were placed in a microtiter plate. The clots were made by the addition of 50μl of thrombin (100U/ml). The ordinate shows OD340 and the abscissa shows incubation time. The turbidity of the clot was measured every 30 min. by a microtiter plate reader with 340 nm of wavelength.

RESULTS

The effects of calcium ion on regular ECLT
Addition of Ca²⁺ to the euglobulin fraction shortened regular ECLT significantly by a factor of 4-5 times in a concentration dependent manner. The significant shortening was observed at 1.5-2.0 mM of Ca²⁺ (Fig.2)

The effects of calcium ion on kaolin activated ECLT
When kaolin was added, ECLT was significantly shortened compared to regular ECLT(Fig.1). In kaolin activated ECLT, however, there was no further shortening by the addition of Ca²⁺ (Data not shown).

The effects of thrombin and calcium ion on regular ECLT
The effect of thrombin concentration on calcium ion induced enhancement of regular ECLT was analyzed The significant shortening of ECLT was observed in all the range of thrombin concentration employed(0-25U/ml), and there was no difference in the extent of the enhancement.

The effects of calcium ion on the plasma clot lysis time
When plasma was used instead of the euglobulin fraction, the addition of Ca²⁺ prolonged the plasma clot lysis time which was initiated by supplementarily added tPA (Fig.3). This prolongation was observed when several different concentrations of tPA were employed (50-200U/ml).

The effects of other divalent cations on regular ECLT
We employed other divalent ions such as Mg^{2+}, Zn^{2+} and Mn^{2+} instead of Ca^{2+}, and those effects on regular ECLT were analyzed. ECLT did not shortened by any other ions except Ca^{2+}. Only Ca^{2+} shortened ECLT(data not shown).

The effects of calcium ion on clot lysis in a purified system
In order to analyze the effects of Ca^{2+} on the degradation of fibrin by plasmin, we employed purified fibrin clot system, which composed of fibrinogen (2μM), Glu-plasminogen (0.5μM), tPA (1U/ml) and thrombin (1U/ml). Clot lysis time in the absence of Ca^{2+} was 190 min. (average of duplicate). and was 220 min. in the presence of Ca^{2+} (16 mM) (average of duplicate). Clot lysis time in the purified system, therefore, did not shorten by the addition of Ca^{2+}.

The effects of calcium on ECLT using barium-absorbed plasma
Barium absorbed plasma was employed in order to see the effects of Ca^{2+}. Regular ECLT of barium absorbed plasma in the absence of Ca^{2+} was 4.3 hours . (average of duplicate) and that in the presence of Ca^{2+} (10 mM) was 1.1 hours (average of duplicate). The significant shortening of regular ECLT was not observed by the addition of Ca^{2+}. Significant shortening by the addition of kaolin with barium absorbed plasma, however, was observed as in the case of normal plasma.

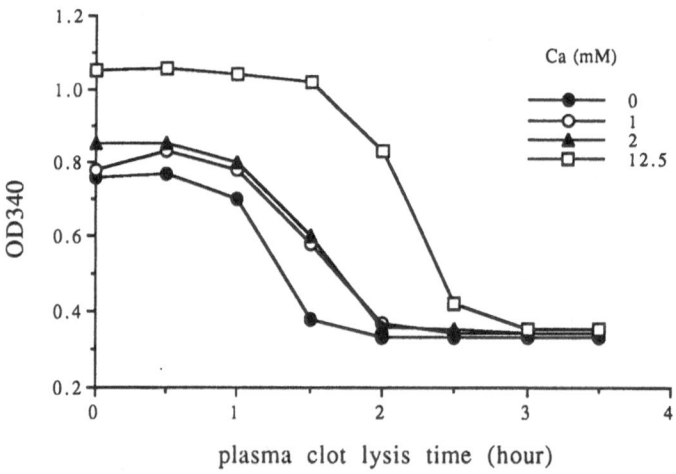

Fig.3 Plasma clot lysis time
100μl of plasma, 50 μl of 50U/ml tPA and 25μl of $CaCl_2$ were placed in a microtiter plate. Clots were made by the addition of 25 μl of thrombin (10U/ml). The turbidity of the clot was measured every 30 min. by the microtiter plate reader with 340nm of wave-length.

DISCUSSION

In the present study, we have shown that in the presence of physiological concentration of Ca^{2+} regular ECLT shortened by a factor of 4-5 times. Shortened ECLT obtained in the presence of Ca^{2+} was similar to kaolin activated ECLT in which intrinsic fibrinolytic pathway is most likely fully activated. These results suggest that Ca^{2+} plays an important role in the activation of fibrinolysis, and that Ca^{2+} may activate the intrinsic pathway. This phenomenon is interesting because it has been believed that Ca^{2+} inhibits fibrinolysis in the plasma system by making fibrin crosslinked and making α_2AP to crosslink to fibrin by activated factor XIII [8]. The calcium dependent enhancement of clot lysis was also not observed in tPA induced plasma clot lysis system in the present study. The enhancement of fibrinolysis by Ca^{2+} seems to be detected only in the euglobulin fraction which contains little amounts of α_2AP. It is, therefore, difficult to know to what extent this calcium dependent enhancement of fibrinolysis is involved in plasma clot lysis.

We then employed a purified system composed of fibrinogen, plasminogen, tPA and thrombin in order to see the effects of Ca^{2+} on fibrin clot lysis. Fibrin clot lysis initiated by tPA was not enhanced by Ca^{2+}. These data suggest that other factors in the euglobulin fraction seem to be involved to enhance ECLT by Ca^{2+}.

In order to know the factors involved in the enhancement, we divided plasma to two fractions by barium absorption technique [9]. In barium-absorbed plasma the shortening of regular ECLT by Ca^{2+} was not observed, which suggests that the factors involved in the enhancement of ECLT by Ca^{2+} is absorbed to barium citrate. Barium citrate absorbed fraction seems to be essential for the enhancement of fibrinolysis by Ca^{2+}.

Since ECLT enhanced by Ca^{2+} was to similar extent to kaolin activated ECLT, it was first suggested that Ca^{2+} may activate intrinsic pathway of fibrinolysis. The fact that the addition of kaolin to barium absorbed plasma shortened ECLT as in normal plasma although Ca^{2+} did not enhance ECLT, however, suggests that the Ca^{2+} dependent enhancement of fibrinolysis is independent of the intrinsic pathway of fibrinolysis. Unknown factors to enhance the activation of fibrinolysis in the euglobulin fraction, therefore, are suggested from our results.

REFERENCES

1. Marsh M (1981) Fibrinolysis. John Wiley & Sons. New York. pp 206- 241

2. Davidson JF, Walker ID (1987) Thromb Haemostas Churchill Livingstone. New York. pp 953-966

3. Urano T, Sumiyoshi K, Pietraszek MH, Takada Y, Takada A (1991) Thromb Haemostas 66 : 474-478

4. Urano T, Sakakibara K, Rydzewski A, Urano S, Takada Y, Takada A (1990) Thromb Haemostas 63 :82-86

5. Carlson RH, Garnick RL, Janes AJS, Meunier AM (1988) Anal Biochem 168 : 428-435

6. Urano S, Metzger AR, Castellino FJ (1989) Proc Nat Acad Sci USA 86 : 2568-2571

7. Deutsch DG and Mertz ET (1970) Science 170 :1095-1096

8. Sakata Y, Aoki N (1982) J. Clin. Invest. 69 : 536-542

9. Bajzar L, Fredenburgh JC, Nesheim M (1990) J Biol Chem 256 : 16948-16954

THE ROLE OF PLATELET PAI-1
IN THE PLATELET RICH PLASMA CLOT LYSIS

K. Serizawa[1], T. Urano[1], Y. Kozima[2], K. Sakakibara[1], Y. Takada[1] and A. Takada[1]

Dept. of Physiology[1] and Medicine[2], Hamamatsu University School of Medicine, Hamamatsu, Shizuoka, JAPAN

Introduction

Plasminogen activator inhibitor-1 (PAI-1) is physiologically the most important inhibitor of tissue plasminogen activator(t-PA) in plasma(1). It has been suggested that more than 80 to 90 % of PAI-1 is stored in the platelet α-granules(2,3). It is not clear, however, whether PAI-1 released from platelet plays an important role in the clot lysis.

Many authors have reported about the specific interactions between platelet and t-PA mediated clot lysis. According to these observations, platelets have been reported to enhance or inhibit fibirinolysis. Several studies suggested that platelets shortened fibrin clot lysis time in vitro, by accelerating plasmin generation on the surface of platelets by t-PA(4,5,6). In contrast, it was also reported that t-PA was less effective to the platelet rich plasma clot(PRP-clot) than to the platelet poor plasma clot(PPP-clot) in vivo(7). However, it is not obvious whether this difference has been induced by the release of PAI-1 from platelet.

We, therefore, investigated the potential role of PAI-1 in platelet by studying the effects of thrombin-activated platelet to the platelet rich plasma clot lysis induced by t-PA.

Materials and Methods

Preparation of PRP and PPP

Blood was collected from the antecubital vein of healthy donors into plastic tubes containing 1/10 volume of 3.8% sodium citrate, pH7.4. To obtain PRP, whole blood was centrifugated at 200 G for 10 min. at 20 °C. The precipitate of PRP was further centrifugated at 1200 G for 10 min. at 4 °C. to obtain PPP. Platelet count in PRP was adjusted to about 30 X 10^4/μl by a dilution with PPP.

Plasma clot lysis assay

96-well microtiter plate was used for the plasma clot lysis assay. 10 μl of human thrombin(10u/ml) was placed in individual wells, followed by the addition of 20μl of two-chain t-PA(30nM) and 70μl of saline. The clot formation was initiated by the addition of 100μl of PRP or PPP preparation, respectively.

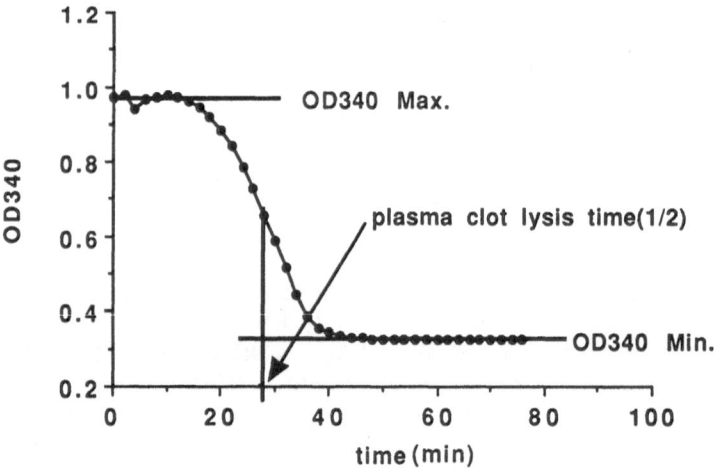

Figure 1. The determination of plasma clot lysis time.
Plasma clot lysis time was determined in microtiter plate reader as written in materials and methods.

The turbidity of the wells, in which plasma clot was made, was measured every 5 minutes employing an automatic microtiter plate reader (Sigma Seiki Inc. Japan). The absorbance data were plotted against time and plasma clot lysis time (1/2) was obtained from the graph as the time which shows the average absorbance of OD 340max and OD 340min(8,9). (Figure 1.)

Antigen levels of PAI-1 in the samples of PR-clot and PP-clot.

After the clots were completely dissolved, we collected the samples and assayed the antigen levels of total PAI-1 and t-PA-PAI-1 complex by enzymeimmuno assay (EIA) as previously described(10,11). Briefly, anti-PAI-1 monoclonal antibody was employed as a first antibody, and anti t-PA polyclonal antibody-β-Galactosidase conjugate was used as a second antibody. The amounts of t-PA-PAI-1 complex were measured in the sample without any pretreatment. In order to measure the amounts of total PAI-1, samples were preincubated with excess amounts of t-PA, and converted all PAI-1 to t-PA-PAI-1 complex. This material was used to assay active total PAI-1. The amounts of free PAI-1 were obtained by the subtraction of the amounts of t-PA-PAI-1 complex from those of total PAI-1. The amounts of free PAI-1 calculated by our method, therefore, arethe amounts of the active form of PAI-1.

Result and Discussion

At first, we compared the t-PA mediated plasma clot lysis time made of PRP and PPP. Fig.2 shows that the lysis time of PRP-clot was longer by 30% than that of PPP-clot. We then made a series of mixed preparations of PRP and PPP. While increasing the relative ratio of PRP in the clot, the lysis time of the clots prolonged. (Fig.2 a, b)

To examine whether this effect was induced by components released from thrombin-activated platelet, prostaglandin E1(PGE1) and theophylline were added to the clots in order to prevent the release and the aggregation of platelets. When PGE1(9mM) and theophylline(450mg/ml) were added to PRP, at which concentration the aggregation of platelets was completely blocked(12)(data not shown), the clot lysis time of PRP shortened almost to that of PPP(Table 1). Table 1 demonstrates that the clot lysis time of PGE1 and theophylline added PR-clot was almost the same as that of PP-clot. These data suggest that the aggregation of platelets plays an important role in the t-PA mediated PR-clot lysis.

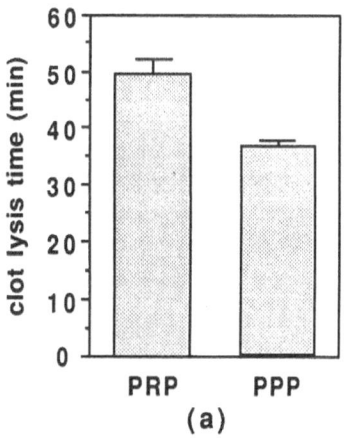

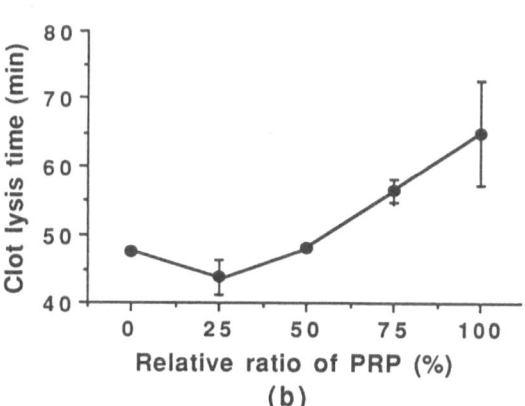

(a)

(b)

Figure 2. (a, b) Effect of platelet on the clot lysis.
(a) t-PA mediated clot lysis time of platelet rich plasma clot (PRP-clot) and of platelet poor plasma clot (PPP-clot).
    In all samples, the lysis time of PRP-clot was longer by 30% than that of PPP-clot.
(b) The relationship between the concentration of platelet and plasma clot lysis time
    We made a series of the mixed preparations of PRP and PPP at different ratios. In proportion to the increase of the relative ratio of PRP in the clot, the lysis time of the clots prolonged.

Table 1. The effect of PGE1 and theophylline on the plasma clot lysis

	CLOT LYSIS TIME (min)	
PGE1&theophylline	(-)	(+)
PRP	49.50±2.65	36.00±1.83
PPP	36.75±0.96	35.50±1.29
		(mean±SE)

Several investigators have reported that PAI-1 existed in platelets has little activity(3,13). They used a method in which residual t-PA activity was measured either by fibrin plate or chromogenic substrate after the addition of t-PA to neutrolyze PAI-1. We then measured the antigen levels of total PAI-1 and t-PA-PAI-1 complex in the samples of PRP-clot and PPP-clot by EIA. In our assay system, only the active form of PAI-1 and t-PA-PAI-1 complex were measured and the amounts of free PAI-1 calculated as previously described are the amounts of active free PAI-1(10,11). Since t-PA was added to initiate clot lysis, most of PAI-1 in PPP existed as tPA-PAI-1-complex. In PRP, however, total PAI-1 was significantly higher than that of PPP and some of them existed as free PAI-1 which possesses activity. When PGE1 and theophylline were used, the antigen levels of total PAI-1 and tPA-PAI-1 complex were essentially the same as PP-clot.

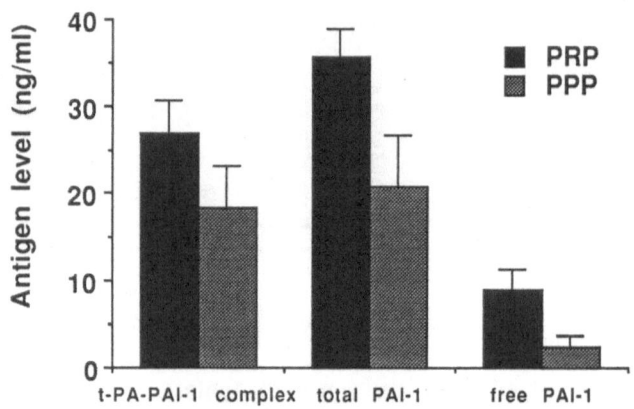

Figure 3. Antigen levels of t-PA-PAI-1 complex, total PAI-1 and free PAI-1 in the samples used for PRP and PPP clot lysis.
In PRP, the amounts of t-PA-PAI-1 complex and total PAI-1 were significantly higher than those in PPP and the amounts of free PAI-1 which possesses activity.were also higher in PRP than PPP.

We therefore concluded that PAI-1 in platelets existed as an active form and PAI-1 released from platelet by thrombin activation effectively inhibited t-PA activity, resulting in the prolongation of plasma clot lysis time. The inhibition of the aggregation and the release of platelets by PGE1 and theophylline successfully prevented the prolongation of clot lysis time of PRP.

Reference

1) Loskufoff,D.J., Sawdey,M. and Mimuro,J.: Coller B.Sed.W.B.Saunders Company, Philladelphia, 87-115.1989.

2) Kruithof,E.K.O , Nicholsa,G. and Bachmann,F.: Blood 70:1645-1653, 1987.

3) Booth,N.A., Simpson,A.J., Croll,A., Bennett,B. and MacGregor,I.R.: British J. Haematology 70:327-333, 1988.

4) Miles,L.A. and Plow,E.F.: J. Biol. Chem. 206:4303-4311, 1985.

5) Vaughan,D.E., Mendelsohn,M.E., Declerck,P.J. von Houtte,E. Collen,D. and Loscalzo,J.: J. Blol. Chem. 264:15869-15874, 1989.

6) Deguchi,K., Murashima,S., Shirakawa,S., Soria,J., Dunn,F. and Tobelem,G.: Thrombos.Res. 40:853-861, 1985.

7) Jang,I.K., Gold,H.K., Zisking,A.A., Fallon,J.T., Holt,R.E., Leinbach,R.C., May,J.W. and Collen,D.: Circulation 79:920-928, 1989.

8) Urano,T., Skakibara,K., Rydzewski A., Urano S., Takada Y. and Takada A.: Thromb Haemostas 63:82-86, 1990.

9) Urano,S., Metzger,A.R.and Castellino,F.J.: Proc Nat Acad Sci USA 86: 2568-2571,.1986.

10) Takada,A., Shizume,K., Ozawa,T., Takahashi,S. and Takada,Y.: Thromb. Res. 42:63-72,1986.

11) Takada.Y. and Takada,A.: Thromb. Res. Suppl. VIII:15-22, 1988.

12) Erickson.,L.A., GInsberg.,M.H. and Loskutoff D.J.: J.Clin.Invest. 74:1465-1472, 1984.

13) Schleef,R.R. Shinha,M. and Loskutoff,D.J.: J. Lab. Clin. Med. 106:408-415, 1985.

THE DISSOCIATION OF α2-PLASMIN-INHIBITOR-PLASMIN COMPLEX TO ACTIVE PLASMIN BY SDS TREATMENT

Dong Yan, Tetsumei Urano, Yumiko Takada and Akikazu Takada

Department of Physiology, Hamamatsu University, School of Medicine, Hamamatsu-shi, Shizuoka-ken 431-31, Japan

INTRODUCTION

α2-PI has been demonstrated to be the physiologically most important inhibitor to plas. in in plasma [1-3], it is a single-chain glycoprotein with molecular weight of about 68,000 [2,4] and inhibits proteolytic activity of plasmin by forming a 1:1 stoichiometric complex which is enzymatically inactive and hardly dissociated by dodecyl sulfate under reducing conditions [5]. α2-PI has been classified as a member of the serine protease inhibitor super family (SERPINS) [6] to which plasminogen activator inhibitor type 1 (PAI-1) also belongs. These protease inhibitors have many similar points in their ways to react with their target enzymes. It has been reported that the complex between PAI-1 and tissue plasminogen activator (t-PA) shows enzymatic activity in zymography [7]. Recently it was also shown that PAI-1 lost its inhibitory activity and was cleaved at the reactive site by PAs after SDS treatment [8]. The latter phenomenon may be responsible for tPA-PAI-1 complex to express enzymatic activity in zymography [8]. Since both PAI-1 and α2-PI are members of SERPINS, it is naturally considered whether SDS has similar effects on α2-PI molecule. We, therefore, investigated the effect of SDS on both α2-PI and α2-PI-plasmin complex in the present study. We also discuss the possible mechanism for α2-PI-plasmin complex to possess enzymatic activity in zymography.

MATERIAL AND METHODS

α2-PI was purified from human plasma according to Müllertz et al [3] and Wiman[9]. The concentration of functionally active α2-PI was determined by titration with plasmin [3]. Plasmin was purchased from KabiVitrum, Stockholm, Sweden. The active site concentration was determined by active site titration with MUGB (4-Methylumbelliferyl p-Guanidinobenzoate), Sigma Chemical company, St. Louis, USA [10]. S-2251 (H-D-Val-Leu-Lys-p-nitroanilide) and fibrinogen were purchased from KABI diagnostica AB, Sweden. Aprotinin (Trasylol) was purchased from Bayer Leverkusen, Germany. Human thrombin was kindly provided by Green Cross, Osaka Japan. SDS-PAGE was done according to Laemmli [11]. Fibrin autography was performed as previously reported [12].

RESULTS

Fibrin autography

Proteolytic activity of plasmin and α2-PI-plasmin complex was analyzed by fibrin autography. α2-PI-plasmin complex was prepared by the incubation of α2-plasmin-inhibitor and plasmin at the molar ratio of 1:0.8 for 30 minutes at room temperature. α2-PI-plasmin complex and plasmin alone were subjected to SDS-PAGE respectively followed by fibrin autography. Fibrinolytic activity was recognized as a lysis zone at the positions of both α2-PI-plasmin complex and plasmin (data not shown).

Effect of SDS on the ability of α2-PI to form a complex with plasmin

The effect of SDS on the ability of α2-PI to form a complex with plasmin was studied. Purified α2-PI(3.35μM) was preincubated with various concentrations of SDS for 30 minutes at room temperature followed by the incubation with the same molar concentration of plasmin(3.32μM) for another 30 minutes. Samples were then subjected to SDS-PAGE and the protein bands were visualized by coomassie blue staining (Fig. 1).

As shown in Figure 1, α2-PI alone showed a single band. Most of α2-PI formed high molecular weight complexes after incubation with plasmin when α2-PI was not pretreated by SDS or treated by 0.001% SDS. When α2-PI was pretreated by 0.1% of SDS, however, the high molecular weight complex band was not observed, and both plasmin and α2-PI migrated to their original positions respectively. In the case of 0.01% SDS, α2-PI did not form complex with plasmin, but was further degraded into a smaller molecule.

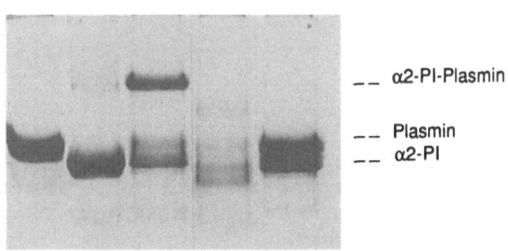

α2-PI-Plasmin

Plasmin
α2-PI

lane 1 lane 2 lane 3 lane 4 lane 5

Figure 1: Effect of SDS on the ability of α2-PI to form a complex with plasmin.
α2-PI was incubated with distilled water (lane 1) or SDS at the final concentrations of 0.001%(lane 2) or 0.01%(lane 3) or 0.1%(lane 4) for 30 minutes, followed by incubation with same molar concentration of plasmin for another 30 minutes. Lane 5 and 6 represent plasmin and α2-PI alone respectively. Proteins were separated by SDS-PAGE and the bands were visualized by coomassie blue staining.

Effect of SDS on the stability of previously formed complex of plasmin and α2-PI

α2-PI-plasmin complex was prepared by incubating the inhibitor and enzyme with a molar ratio of 1.0 to 0.8 at room temperature for 30 minutes. SDS at final concentrations of 0.1%, 0.01% and 0.001% was added to the mixtures and the activity of dissociated plasmin was monitored by the release of paranitroaniline using microtiter plate reader (Bioreader FS-340, Sigma company, Japan) at the wavelength of 405 nm. As shown in Figure 2, when α2-PI-plasmin complex was treated by 0.1% and 0.01% SDS, the mixture showed obvious hydrolysis of the substrate S-2251. In contrast, when α2-PI-plasmin complex was not treated by SDS or treated by 0.001% SDS, no hydrolysis of S-2251 was observed. Hydrolysis of S-2251 by SDS treated α2-PI-plasmin complex at the concentrations of 0.1% or 0.01% was completely abolished by the addition of aprotinin at the concentration of 3000u/ml(data not shown), suggesting that the hydrolysis was initiated by plasmin which was most likely generated by the dissociation of α2-PI-plasmin complex induced by SDS treatment.

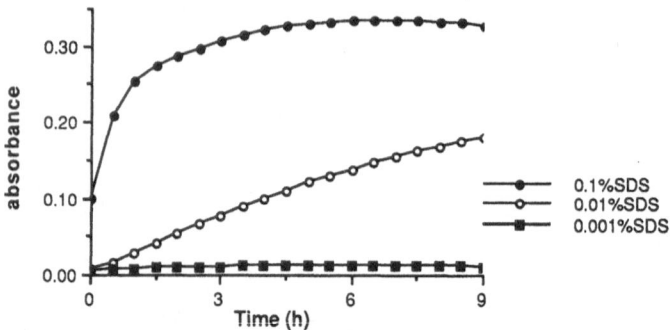

Figure 2: Detection of dissociated plasmin's activity by SDS treatment of α2-PI-plasmin complex with S-2251.
α2-PI-plasmin complex was preincubated either with SDS at the final concentrations of 0.1%, 0.01%, or 0.001% for 30 minutes. The activity of dissociated plasmin was then monitored by the hydrolysis of S-2251(final concentration of 100 µg/ml) at a wave length of 405 nm.

DISCUSSION

In the present study, we demonstrated that α2-PI-plasmin complex could be dissociated by the treatment with SDS, releasing the free active form of plasmin and that this finding may explain the possible mechanism for α2-PI-plasmin complex to express protease activity in zymography after SDS-PAGE.

When α2-PI was treated by 0,1% SDS, it lost its inhibitory ability toward plasmin by forming a high molecular weight complex. Since the amidolytic activity of plasmin was not affected by SDS treatment, this functional change was likely caused by conformational change of α2-PI induced by SDS. When α2-PI was treated by 0.01% SDS, dramatic change happened. α2-PI not only lost its ability to inhibit plasmin by forming a high molecular weight complex, but was cleaved into a lower molecular weight form by plasmin. These results suggest that α2-PI may adopt at least three different types of conformation. One is an intact form which possesses activity to form a complex with plasmin. The second form can be obtained by the treatment of 0.1% SDS and has no activity to form a complex with plasmin. The third form, which can be induced by 0.01% SDS treatment, is a substrate-like form that has no activity but can be cleaved into smaller molecules by plasmin.

These characteristics seem to be similar to those of PAI-1 as reported recently [8]. It was shown that treatment of PAI-1 by 0.01% SDS changed its conformation resulting in the disappearance of the inhibitory activity against its target proteases, plasminogen activators. At the concentration of 0.1%, SDS treatment changed the function of PAI-1 totally converting an inhibitor of plasminogen activators to a substrate of those proteases which was easily cleaved at its reactive site. Such alteration of both function and conformation by SDS treatment, therefore, may be a common characteristic of the SERPINS to which both α2-PI and PAI-1 belong.

We then investigated the effect of SDS on the complex between α2-PI and plasmin. The incubation of previously prepared α2-PI-plasmin complex with different concentrations of SDS dissociated the complex, releasing free plasmin of which the activity was detected by S-2251. This activity was quenched completely by aprotinin. These results conflict by S-2251. This activity was quenched completely by aprotinin. These results conflict with the previous data which have shown that high molecular weight complex between serine protease and the SERPINS was highly stable and was not dissociated by SDS-PAGE[7]. Many lines of data, however, have shown that the specific activity of serine protease could be detected at the position of high molecular weight complex with the SERPINS in zymography after SDS-PAGE[7,8], which suggest that the protease recovered its specific activity either by being dissociated from the complex or by the alteration of the conformation of the reactive site of the SERPINS. From the data of the present study, we may consider the mechanism for this phenomenon as follows. When the complex between plasmin and α2-PI was exposed to SDS during SDS-PAGE, plasmin could be dissociated from the complex and expressed its specific activity on fibrin autography. The release of free plasmin from the complex by SDS treatment, therefore, may be responsible for the expression of proteolytic activity in fibrin zymography or casein zymography. Another possibility, however, that the exposure of the active site of plasmin in the complex without complete dissociation is responsible for the expression of protease activity may not be negligible.

The interaction between plasmin and α2-PI occurs initially between a lysine binding site(s) of plasmin and a complementary site in α2-PI, which is responsible for the first step of reversible reaction. The second step follows by a reaction between the active site serine of plasmin and the reactive site of α2-PI, which is responsible for the irreversible reaction [13,14]. It is of interest, however, that not only the reversible complex but the previously formed irreversible complex was dissociated by SDS treatment releasing the intact form of plasmin. We believe that the present work will contribute to the analysis of the mechanism of the interaction between the SERPINS and serine proteases.

REFERENCES

1. Collen D (1976) Eur J Biochem 69: 209-216

2. Moroi M, Aoki N (1976) J Biol Chem 251: 5956-5965

3. Müllertz S, Clemmensen I (1976) Biochem J 159: 545-553

4. Wiman B, Collen D (1977) Eur J Biochem 78: 19-26

5. Wiman B, Collen D (1979) J Biol Chem 254: 9291-9297

6. Carrell R (1984) Nature 312: 14

7. Takada Y, Takada A (1991) Thrombosis Research 63: 169-177

8. Urano T, Strandberg L, Johansson B-AL, Ny T (1992) Eur J Biochem in press.

9. Wiman B (1980) Biochem J 191: 229-232

10. Jameson GW, Roberts DV, Adams RW, Kyle WSA, Elmore DT (1973) Biochem J 131: 107-117

11. Laemmli KU (1970) Nature 227: 680-685

12. Granelli-piperno A, Reich M (1978) J Exp Med 148: 223-234

13. Christensen U, Clemmensen I (1977) Biochem J 163: 389-391

14. Wiman B, Collen D (1978) Eur J Biochem 84: 573-578

Platelets and antithrombotic agents

COLLAGEN-INDUCED PLATELET AGGREGATION WAS MIMICKED BY SNAKE VENOM PROTEIN AND INHIBITED BY PLANT COMPONENT

Che-Ming Teng, Feng-Nien Ko, Chien-Huan Lin and *Chung-Nan Lin

Pharmacological Institute, College of Medicine, National Taiwan University, Taipei and *School of Pharmacy, Kaohsiung Medical College, Kaohsiung, Taiwan.

KEY WORDS: Collagen, Trimucytin, Frangulin B, Platelet Aggregation.

ABSTRACT

Trimucytin is a potent ($EC_{50} = 0.8$ nM) platelet aggregation inducer isolated from *Trimeresurus mucrosquamatus* snake venom. The aggregation was independent of ADP, thromboxane or PAF pathway. Forskolin and sodium nitroprusside inhibited both platelet aggregation and ATP release. In quin-2-loaded platelets, intracellular Ca^{2+} concentration raised by trimucytin was decreased by 12-O-tetradecanoyl phorbol-13 acetate, imipramine, TMB-8 and indomethacin. Inositol phosphate formation in platelets was markedly enhanced by both trimucytin and collagen. MAB 1988, an antibody against platelet membrane glycoprotein Ia, inhibited trimucytin and collagen-induced platelet aggregation and ATP release. Frangulin B, an emodin glycoside, was isolated from plant *Rhamus formosana*. It inhibited selectively collagen- and trimucytin-induced shape change, aggregation, ATP release and thromboxane formation of platelets, without affecting those induced by arachidonic acid, ADP, PAF and thrombin. Similarly, the formation of inositol phosphate caused by collagen was also suppressed by frangulin B, while those by PAF and thrombin were not affected. Frangulin B also decreased Mg^{2+}-dependent platelet adhesion to collagen. It is concluded that trimucytin may activate collagen receptors on platelet membrane, and causes aggregation and release reaction mainly through phospholipase C-phosphoinositide pathway, while frangulin B may be an antagonist of collagen receptors.

INTRODUCTION

Following injury to the blood vessel wall, components under the vessel wall are brought into contact with the circulating blood. Among these, collagen fibers are the most important. Adhesion of platelets to the pre-exposed collagen is the first step in the hemostatic process. Subsequent platelet aggregation and plug formation are responsible for the arrest of bleeding [1]. Platelet-collagen interaction may also take important roles in pathological thrombus formation [2].

Platelet adhesion and aggregation in the presence of collagen have been studied in many laboratories. It is well accepted that platelet membrane glycoprotein Ia/IIa complex may be the receptors mediating collagen activation of platelets. The complex is a member of the integrin family of adhesive protein receptors with the 160 KDa subunit designed the α_2 chain and the 130 KDa subunit designed the β_1 chain [3,4].

Snake venoms can affect platelet functions in various ways. Some induced platelet aggregation and release reaction while other inhibit these processes. Many active proteins have been purified recently [5]. In oriental traditional medicine, a lots of herbal drugs have been claimed to possess "antithrombotic-vasoactive" effects. In recent years, we have studied and isolated some antiplatelet agents from herbal plants [6]. In this paper, we reported a snake venom protein which mimicked collagen activation of platelets and a herbal component which might inhibit platelet aggregation and adhesion through the collagen receptors.

MATERIALS AND METHODS

Materials

Trimucytin was purified from *Trimeresurus mucrosquamatus* snake venom [7]. Frangulin B was isolated from *Rhamnus formosana* [8]. Collagen obtained from Sigma Chem. Co. U.S.A. was homogenized in 25 mM acetic acid and then stored at -70°C. Thrombin (bovine) was obtained from Park Davis Co. U.S.A. MAB 1988 was purchased from Chemicon International Inc., U.S.A. Kadsurenone was kindly supplied by Merck, Sharp and Dohme, U.S.A. Quin-2 AM and myo-[2-^{3}H]inositol were purchased from Amersham Lab., England. Thromboxane B_2 RIA kits were obtained from New England Nuclear Co., U.S.A. Arachidonic acid, ADP, platelet-activating factor (PAF), 12-O-tetradecanoyl phorbol-13-acetate (TPA), sodium nitroprusside, forskolin, TMB-8, creatine phosphate and creatine phosphokinase were purchased from Sigma Chem. Co. U.S.A.

Platelet functional tests

Washed rabbit platelets were prepared as described by Ardlie *et al.* [9] and suspended in Tyrode's solution containing 1 mM of calcium and 0.35% of bovine serum albumin. Aggregation was measured by the turbidimetric method of Born and Cross [10] and the percent aggregation was calculated as described previously [11]. ATP released from platelets was detected by bioluminescence method as described by DeLuca and McElory [12]. Measurement was performed at 37°C, 1200 rpm stirring, and recorded with a Lumi- aggregometer (Chrono-Log Co., U.S.A.). Thromboxane B_2 was measured after EDTA (2 mM) and indomethacin (50 μM) were added to platelet suspension 6 min after the addition of inducers using radioimmunoassay kits (New England Nuclear, U.S.A.). Measurement of phosphoinositide breakdown using inositol monophosphate as an indicator was modified from those of Huang and Detwiler [13] and Neylon and Summers [14]. Intracellular calcium was measured by the method of Rink *et al.* [15] using quin-2 loaded platelets. Platelet adhesion to collagen was measured by the methods of Santoro [3] and Coller *et al.* [16].

RESULTS AND DISCUSSION

Platelet Aggregation Induced by Trimucytin

Trimucytin, isolated from the snake venom of *T. mucrosquamatus*, is a glycoprotein with a molecular weight of 68 KDa. It initiated the aggregation and ATP release of washed rabbit platelets at a concentration as low as 10 ng/ml. At 1 μg/ml, it caused platelet aggregation to a similar extent (80-90% aggregation) as 100 μM arachidonic acid or 10 μg/ml collagen.

ADP is an important endogenous mediator released from dense bodies of platelets [17]. Trimucytin (1 μg/ml)-induced platelet aggregation (90.5$\pm$1.8%, n=4) was not significantly suppressed by ADP-scavenger, creatine phosphate/creatine phosphokinase (CP/CPK, 5 mM/8U/ml) (88.4$\pm$3.5%, n=4), or PAF antagonist, kadsurenone (30 μM) (90.6$\pm$3.7, n=4). Indomethacin (10-50 μM) inhibited only the thromboxane B_2 formation, but not the aggregation caused by trimucytin or collagen. These data indicate that trimucytin-induced aggregation is not dependent on ADP release, thromboxane or PAF formation in rabbit platelets. Forskolin (20 μM) and sodium nitroprusside (10 μM) abolished completely the ATP release from platelets, and inhibited markedly the aggregation but not the shape change induced by trimucytin.

In addition to aggregation and ATP release, trimucytin caused a rapid increase of the intracellular calcium, $[Ca^{2+}]_i$, of quin-2 loaded rabbit platelets. Pretreatment of indomethacin (50 μM) decreased this $[Ca^{2+}]_i$ rise, but not the aggregation, while pretreatment of imipramine (100 μM) and TMB-8 (10 μM) decreased this $[Ca^{2+}]_i$ rise profoundly and completely blocked the aggregation. A phorbol ester (12-O-tetradecanoyl phorbol-13-acetate, TPA) also showed inhibition on both the aggregation and rise of $[Ca^{2+}]_i$ caused by trimucytin (1 μg/ml).

In the presence of calcium (1 mM) and indomethacin (50 μM), collagen (10 μg/ml) and trimucytin (1 and 10 μg/ml) respectively caused 7.3$\pm$1.8, 7.2$\pm$1.8 and 21.9$\pm$6.9 folds of the increase of inositol monophosphate formation compared with the resting level.

MAB 1988 is a mouse monoclonal antibody against human platelet membrane glycoprotein Ia [18]. At 10 μg/ml, MAB 1988 inhibited markedly collagen (10 μg/ml)-induced platelet aggregation and ATP release reaction. The responses of platelets to trimucytin (1 μg/ml) were almost completely suppressed by MAB 1988 (10 μg/ml). However, increase of the concentration of trimucytin (2-20 μg/ml) could overcome this inhibition.

Antiplatelet Action of Frangulin B

Frangulin B (10-100 μg/ml), a glycoside derivative of emodin, inhibited selectively and concentration-dependently the platelet aggregation and ATP release induced by collagen, but not that by arachidonic acid (100 μM), ADP (20 μM), PAF (2 ng/ml) or thrombin (0.1 U/ml) even at a concentration as high as 100 μg/ml which showed complete inhibition on collagen-induced platelet aggregation. Incubation of frangulin B with platelets for 30 min did not cause a more pronouced inhibition than that for 3 min, and the inhibitory effect of frangulin B on platelet aggregation could be washed out and the aggregability of platelets was restored. Shape change of platelets caused by collagen was not affected while both aggregation and ATP release were completely inhibited. Similar inhibition could be observed in trimucytin (1 μg/ml)-induced platelet aggregation and ATP release. Both concentration-inhibition curves of frangulin B against collagen- and trimucytin-induced platelet aggregation are parallel and the IC_{50} values are calculated to be about 30 and 12 μg/ml, respectively.

Thromboxane B_2 formation in washed rabbit platelets challenged with collagen (10 μg/ml), arachidonic acid (100 μM) or thrombin (0.1 U/ml) for 6 min was measured.   Frangulin B showed concentration-dependent inhibition on the thromboxane B_2 formation caused by collagen, without affecting that by arachidonic acid or thrombin.   ADP or PAF did not cause thromboxane B_2 formation in rabbit platelets [20,21], thus the thromboxane B_2 formation in ADP- or PAF-treated platelets was not studied.

Phosphoinositide breakdown was observed in platelets activated by many agonists [22,23]. In this study, we found collagen, PAF and thrombin induced inositol monophosphate formation. Only the formation of inositol monophosphate caused by collagen, but not PAF or thrombin, was decreased by frangulin B.

Collagen or bovine serum albumin was coated in polystyrene microtiter wells, and washed rabbit platelets were added and allowed to adhere for 30 min at 22°C. Platelets adhered to collagen with a density of 126 ± 18 platelets/mm^2, while to bovine serum albumin of 17 ± 12 platelets/mm^2. If frangulin B (25,50 μg/ml) was presented, only 80 ± 10 and 47 ± 7 platelets/mm^2 were adhered to collagen, respectively. The percent inhibitions were calculated to be 36.5 and 62.6% for 25 and 50 μg/ml of frangulin B, respectively.

In this paper, we found a snake venom protein trimucytin possessed very potent aggregating activity. The action was proposed to be the activation of collagen-receptors on platelet membrane because it can be inhibited selectively by the monoclonal antibody of glycoprotein Ia. We also found a plant component frangulin B inhibited selectively collagen- and trimucytin-induced platelet aggregation. The signal transduction after collagen activation of platelet membrane receptors was also suppressed. Thus, both agents may be valuable research tools for the study of collagen-platelet interaction.

Acknowledgements

This work was supported by research grants of the National Science Council of the Republic of China (NSC78-0412-B002-60 and NSC81-0412-B002-113).

REFERENCES

1. Baumgartner HR (1977) Thrombos Hemostas 37: 1-16

2. Santoro SA, Cunningham LW (1981) In: Gorden JL (ed) Platelets in Biology and Pathology 2, Elsevier/Amsterdam pp 249-264

3. Santoro SA (1986) Cell 46: 913-920

4. Hemler ME, Huang C, Schwarz L (1987) J Biol Chem 262: 3300-3309

5. Teng CM, Huang TF (1991) Platelets 2: 1-11

6. Teng CM, Ko FN, Wang JP, Lin CN, Wu TS, Chen CC, Huang TF (1991) J Pharm Pharmacol 43: 667-669

7. Ouyang C, Wang JP, Teng CM (1980) Biochim Biophys Acta 630: 246-253

8. Lin CN, Chung MI, Lu CM (1990) Phytochem 29: 3903-3905

9. Ardlie NG, Perry DW, Packham MA, Mustard JF (1971) Proc Soc Exp Biol Med 136: 1021-1023

10. Born GVR, Cross MJ (1963) J Physiol 168: 178-195

11. Teng CM, Ko FN (1988) Thrombos Hemostas 59: 304-309

12. DeLuca M, McElory WD (1978) Method Enzymol 57: 3-15

13. Huang EM, Detwiler TC (1986) Biochem J 236: 895-901

14. Neylon CB, Summers RJ (1987) Br J Pharmacol 91: 367-373

15. Rink TJ, Sanchez A, Hallam TJ (1983) Nature 305: 317-319

16. Coller BB, Beer JH, Scudder LE, Steinberg MH (1989) Blood 74: 182-192

17. Packham MA, Guccione MA, Greenberg JP, Kinlough-Rathobone RL, Mustard JF (1977) Blood 50: 915-926

18. Staatz WD, Rajpara SM, Wayner EA, Carter WG, Santoro SA J (1989) Cell Biol 108: 1917-1924

19. Teng CM, Hung ML, Ko FN, Tsai IH, Huang TF (1993) Thrombos Hemostas (in press)

20. Teng CM, Chen WY, Ko WC, Ouyang C (1987) Biochim Biophys Acta 24 375-382

21. Lazenave JP, Benveniste J, Mustard JF (1979) Lab Invest 41: 275-285

22. Broekman MJ, Ward JW, Marcus AJ (1980) J Clin Invest 66: 275-283

23. Billah MM, Lapetina EG (1982) J Biol Chem 257: 5196-5200

ANTIPLATELET ACTIVITY OF A THROMBIN-LIKE ENZYME IN EXPERIMENTAL RABBITS

Tur-Fu Huang and Mei-Chi Chang

Pharmacological Institute, College of Medicine,
National Taiwan University, Taipei, Taiwan.

KEY WORDS: Thrombin-like enzyme, antiplatelet function, defibrinogenation, fibrin/fibrinogen degradation products.

ABSTRACT

Thrombin-like enzyme (TLE) has been utilized for the prevention of venous thromboembolism because of its rapid defibrinogenating effect *in vivo*. However, there are still conflicting reports concerning with its effect on platelet function. In this report, TLE purified from venom of *Calloselasma rhodostoma* was administered to rabbits intravenously, blood samples prior to or 1,3,6 and 24 hours after infusion were taken for assays. TLE caused a rapid and sustained defibrinogenation within the first 1-6 hour, and production of fibrin/fibrinogen degradation products (FDPs) peaking at 1 hour and declining to control level at 6-hour. However, no significant changes were found with platelet count, white cell count and hematocrit value. Citrated platelet-rich plasma (PRP) prepared at 1,3 and 6 hours after TLE infusion showed a diminished activity in aggregation, ATP release and thromboxane B_2 formation upon the addition of collagen. However, platelet suspension prepared from defibrinogenated PRP at 3-hour showed a normal aggregation and ATP-releasing activity. When the remaining plasma was used to suspend the normal platelets prepared from PRP prior to TLE treatment, the platelets showed a similar defect in aggregation and release reaction. Addition of fibrinogen (200 μg/ml) partially restored aggregation activity but not the capacity of secretion and thromboxane formation. 6-Ketoprostaglandin $F_{1\alpha}$, the metabolite of PGI_2, was significantly increased and the viscosity of the whole blood was decreased at 6-hour after infusion. In summary, we confirmed the antiplatelet function of TLE *ex vivo* and suggest that the sustained defibrinogenation is the primary cause leading to the impairment of platelet function after TLE infusion. On the other hand, the production of fibrin/fibrinogen degradation products at the initial stage may also be involved. The reduced blood viscosity and the enhancement of PGI_2 levels are beneficial for thromboembolic disorder.

INTRODUCTION

Ancrod (Arvin) is the thrombin-like enzyme purified from the venom of malayan pit viper. Through the breakdown of plasma fibrinogen and formation of fibrin monomers, it causes rapid defibrinogenation.[1] It selectively cleaves fibrinopeptide A of fibrinogen.[2] In the urokinase sensitivity test system, clots formed by the action of ancrod were not cross-linked and were more susceptible to the lytic action of exogenous plasmic action than the comparable thrombin clots.[3] The clots were rapidly removed from the circulation, either by fibrinolysis or through phagocytosis by cells of the reticulo-endothelial system.[4,5]

Defibrinogenation has influence on the rate of disappearance of pre-formed thrombi in clinical[6,7] and experimental conditions.[8] Thrombin-like enzyme (TLE) has been used in several clinical conditions, such as intermittent claudication,[9] in the prevention of deep vein thrombosis and thrombo-embolic condition,[10] in extracorporeal circulation systems,[11] and in protecting venous grafts[12,13] or arterial grafts.[1] It has also been used in patients with peripheral arterial occlusive disease to prevent the reoccurance of thrombosis after successful thrombolysis.[14]

Ancrod has no direct effect on the coagulation system other than fibrinogen.[15,16] It does not directly activate plasminogen.[3] At the same time, ancrod had little effect on platelet aggregation *in vitro* and no effect on platelet survival *in vivo*.[17,18] However, early reports of *in vitro* aggregation of platelets from subjects who have received parental ancrod have been conflicting. Some reported no change[6,7] while others reported transient inhibition of aggregation.[18-20] However, one group found a negative correlation between aggregation and serum fibrin degradation product titers and a positive correlation aggregation and plasma fibrinogen concentration[19] whereas the other reported that aggregation was independent of fibrinogen concentration[18]. In view of above reports, ancrod is a potential therapeutic agent in prevention and treatment of thrombosis. However, there is no consistent data indicating that its therapeutic effect is related to its effect on platelet function *in vivo*.

The purpose of this paper is to examine if any impairment of platelet function occurs following the intravenous infusion of thrombin- like enzyme in experimental rabbits and to investigate its possible mechanism of action. In addition to defibrinogenating effect, the production of FDPs, elevated PGI_2 and reduced blood viscosity were observed. In viewing of these results, we conclude that the sustained defibrinogenating effect is the key factor responsible for its antiplatelet effect *ex vivo* while other changes are complimentary to its antiplatelet action.

MATERIALS AND METHODS

Materials

Thrombin-like enzyme (TLE) was purified from the venom of *Calloselasma rhodostoma*. It was eluted as a single homogenous peak on the analytical high-performance liquid chromatography (HPLC) gel filtration column (PROTEIN PAK 300 sw, Waters) and it contains only one N-terminal amino acid residue, valine. The TLE selectively cleaved fibrinopeptide A of fibrinogen as shown by reverse-phase HPLC. The specific activity (NIH units) of this purified TLE was calculated to be around 1,000 U/mg according to defined method of Seegers, 1962. Elisa kits of 6-keto prostaglandin $F_{1\alpha}$ (6-keto $PGF_{1\alpha}$), thromboxane B_2 (TXB_2) were purchased from Cayman Chem. Co.. A kit for detection of fibrin/fibrinogen degradation products (FDPs) was purchased from DIAGNOSTICA STAGO. Collagen (type I, bovine achilles tendon), obtained from Sigma Chemical Co., was homogenized in 25 mM acetic acid and stored at -70°C at a concentration of 1 mg/ml. Unless otherwise mentioned, all other chemicals were purchased from Sigma Chemical Co..

Experimental Animals

Rabbits of either sex weighing 2-2.5 kg were used in these studies. TLE dissolved in 3 ml saline at doses of 0.3, 0.5 or 1 unit per kg of body weight was infused for 30 minutes by a constant-infusion pump. Blood samples were drawn from marginal ear vein at the indicated time intervals. One milliliter of blood was placed in a glass tube for determination of the whole blood clotting time[22] or mixed with a mixture of indomethacin (200 μM), EDTA (5 mM), heparin (50 U/ml) and aprotinin (100 g/ml) for the determination of 6-keto $PGF_{1\alpha}$ and FDPs. However, blood samples for platelet aggregation tests were collected in plastic tubes containing 3.8% sodium citrate and mixed at a ratio of 9:1 (v/v). The Brookfield viscometer (model LVTDV-II) was used to measure the viscosity of whole blood.

Plasma Fibrinogen Concentration

Plasma fibrinogen level was estimated by fibrinogen assay system (Fibriquik, Organon Teknika) based on the Clauss method.[23]

Fibrin/Fibrinogen Degradation Products (FDPs)

FDPs was detected semi-quantitatively by agglutination of latex particles coated with specific antibodies for fragments D and E.

6-Keto-Prostaglandin $F_{1\alpha}$ and Thromboxane B_2 Formation

The 6-keto $PGF_{1\alpha}$ of plasma and TXB_2 formation of platelets in PRP were measured by using the Elisa kit according to instruction of the manufacturer.

Platelet Function Test

Platelet-rich plasma (PRP) was prepared from whole blood anticoagulated with sodium citrate (9:1, v/v) and centrifuged at 90 xg for 10 minutes. *Ex vivo* platelet aggregability of PRP was measured at 37°C by the turbidimetric method.[24] Aggregation was induced by ADP and collagen at a final concentration of 20 μM and 10 μg/ml, respectively. The aggregation response was measured as the maximal change of light absorbance as compared to platelet- poor plasma (PPP) and expressed as % aggregation. ATP released from platelets was detected by the bioluminescence method[25] using luciferin/luciferase mixture (20 μl). In further experiments, the effect of citrated plasma from TLE treated rabbits on the aggregation of normal washed platelets was investigated. The platelet suspension was obtained from EDTA-anticoagulated PRP according to the washing procedure described previously[26]. The platelet pellets were finally suspended in citrated plasma obtained from rabbit at different time-intervals prior to or after TLE infusion, and platelet number was counted by Coulter Counter (Model ZM), adjusted to 3×10^8 platelets per milliliter. This citrated plasma used to resuspend the washed platelets was generally kept at room temperature longer than one hour in order to exclude the possible involvement of PGI_2 factor.[27]

Statistical Analysis

Statistical significance was determined by the Student *t* test; a *p* value of < 0.05 was chosen to denote statistical significance between control and experimental groups. Unless indicated otherwise, the data are presented as mean$\pm$SEM (n).

RESULTS

Blood Behaviour of Defibrinogenation

There was no statistically significant changes in platelet count, white cell count or haematocrit value after TLE infusion (1 U/kg) (data not shown). However, there was a significant decrease in blood viscosity at shear rates tested 6 hours after TLE infusion (0.5 U/kg), it returned to normal level 24 hours after TLE treatment (exception at shear rate $23.0 \, s^{-1}$) (Table 1). The whole blood was rendered incoagulable after TLE infusion and its coagulability returned to normal within 24 hours after TLE administration.

Effect on Platelet Aggregation

TLE even at a concentration higher than 50 U/ml, exerted no significant on aggregation of washed platelets *in vitro*. However, it exhibited inhibitory effect on platelet aggregation when given intravenously. Its inhibitory effect on platelet aggregation and ATP release induced by ADP ($20 \, \mu M$), collagen ($10 \, \mu g/ml$) or PAF ($2 \, ng/ml$) peaked at 3-hour and lasted for more than 9 hours after intravenous infusion of TLE at doses tested (0.3, 0.5 and 1 U/kg), and completely waned within 24 hours. It was found that platelet aggregation as well as thromboxane formation induced by collagen was inhibited at 1,3 and 6 hours after TLE infusion. However, both aggregation and thromboxane B_2 formation of PRP restored to normal after 24 hours. When platelet suspension prepared from the defibrinogenated blood (at 6-hour) showed normal aggregation and ATP release induced by collagen ($10 \, \mu g/ml$) (data not shown). The platelet aggregability after defibrinogenation could be recovered by washing platelets with Tyrode solution. This indicated that platelets themselves were apparently functionally intact ever after TLE treatment. Therefore, we further investigated how the reduced aggregability of platelets in the defibrinogenated plasma was caused.

The Relationship of Fibrinogen, FDPs Level and Platelet Aggregation

The experimental results obtained from different doses tested (0.3, 0.5 and 1 U/kg) all showed that the reduced platelet aggregation correlated very well with the reduction of fibrinogen level throughout the experimental time course. It was also noted that the fall in fibrinogen level was immediately accompanied by a rise in FDPs which is an indirect index of the activation of the fibrinolytic system *in vivo*. FDPs level were highest at 1 hour and returned to resting level at 6 hours after TLE infusion (1.0 U/kg). However, the platelet function of PRP obtained at 6-hour was only partially restored (12.7% of control).

PGI$_2$ Levels After Thrombin-Like Enzyme Infusion

6-Keto PGF$_{1\alpha}$ (PGI$_2$ stable metabolite) level of plasma was significantly elevated at 6-hour after the infusion of TLE (1.0 U/kg) (279.5 ± 17.9 vs 172.2 ± 34.1 pg/ml).

Effect of the Citrated Plasma from Defibrinogenated Rabbit on Platelet Function of the Normal Washed Platelets

In the following experiments, we examined the effect of the citrated plasma obtained from 0 and 3-hour after TLE infusion, which was kept at room temperature at least one hour for ruling out the PGI$_2$ effect on platelet function of washed platelets of normal rabbit. The inhibitory effect on platelet aggregation varied when the volume ratio of citrated plasmas (0 hour: 3-hour) changed. It was found that the smaller the ratio, the lesser degree of platelet aggregation caused by collagen was observed. When the washed platelets were simply suspended with the defibrinogenated citrated plasma at 3-hour, % aggregation was significantly reduced ($13.3 \pm 2.3\%$ vs. $85.2 \pm 2.0\%$, $p < 0.001$). In the meantime, the thromboxane B_2 formation of platelets stimulated by collagen was decreased in parallel. It was noted that the platelet aggregation in the citrated plasma at a volumn ratio of 0:4 (0 hour: 3 -hour) was greatly reduced when compared with that in plasma at a ratio of 1:3 (13.3% vs. 68.0%, respectively). The fibrinogen level in plasma at the ratio of 1:3 was about 500 $\mu g/ml$ which was usually sufficient for supporting platelet aggregation in the preparation of platelet suspension. Under the same condition, when fibrinogen was added to the defibrinogenated plasma at a final concentration of 200 $\mu g/ml$, % aggregation was increased from 11.3 ± 2.3 to $50.1 \pm 9.6\%$ while the reduced thromboxane B_2 formation and ATP release were unchanged even after the addition of fibrinogen. However, a further increase of fibrinogen concentration above 200 $\mu g/ml$ did not enhance platelet aggregation any further. In addition, the addition of aprotinin (100 KIU/ml) to this defibrinogenated plasma prior to suspending the washed normal platelets had no effect on platelet aggregation or ATP release, indicating that the impairment of platelet function was not caused by plasmin existing in plasma.

DISCUSSION

The importance of platelets in hemostasis and thrombosis is generally recognized. Therefore, the reduced platelet aggregation may increase the therapeutic effect of anticoagulants in the prevention of relapse of thrombosis by inhibiting the deposition of platelets on the existing thrombus. There was an impaired aggregation response to ADP occurring one hour after the start of TLE infusion to rabbits. This pattern of the impaired aggregation response to TLE infusion was also observed when platelets were challenged by collagen or PAF. This was corresponding to the reduced platelet aggregability with batroxobin (a thrombin-like enzyme purified from *Bothrops atrox* venom) treated patients[28,29] and ancrod experiments.[18-20] However, platelet survival and platelet counts in ancrod treated rabbits were normal.[17] In addition, washed platelets prepared from the defibrinogenated rabbits retained their ability of aggregation and ATP release in response to collagen. Platelet function of the defibrinogenated PRP was restored by washing after removing inhibitor(s) of platelets present in plasma. It had been reported that a negative correlation between aggregation and serum FDPs.[18,19] Previous reports demonstrated that FDPs inhibited platelet aggregation,[30-32] platelet serotonin release induced by thrombin.[31] There are two possible explanations for the inhibitory effects of FDPs on aggregation; firstly the competition for the fibrinogen receptor by FDPs which are unable to support aggregation[33,34] or secondly the binding of FDPs to fibrinogen, leading to impairment of fibrinogen binding to platelet surface.[35,36] However, our results indicated that FDPs level increased immediately after the reduction of fibrinogen level (at 1 and 3 hours after TLE infusion) reflecting the activation of endogenous fibrinolytic system. These results were consistent with the reported reduction of plasminogen level after ancrod administration.[37,38] FDPs level but not platelet aggregability returned to normal level at 6 hours of experimental time course. Therefore, factor(s) other than FDPs may impair platelet function of the defibrinogenated animals. In this study, platelet function of PRP from the TLE treated rabbits was well correlated with plasma fibrinogen concentration through the full time course. The addition of exogenous fibrinogen partially restored aggregation of normal platelets suspended in defibrinogenated plasmas. This is in accordance with the report of Gouin *et al.*[39] that platelet function of washed platelets suspended in plasma depleted of fibrinogen could be partially restored to control by addition of fibrinogen. Like previous reports,[39-43] we presumed trace amounts of fibrinogen seem to be essential for normal aggregation in plasma. As shown in Table 3, the addition of exogenous fibrinogen partially restored platelet aggregation whereas it caused no significant increase of thromboxane formation of platelets. It had been demonstrated that a specific fibrinogen antagonist had no significant effect on thromboxane B_2 formation of platelets stimulated by thrombin.[44] The impairment of platelets in releasing mechanism may indicate that factor(s) other than the reduction of fibrinogen may be involved.

In addition to the elevation of FDPs and the reduced fibrinogen level of plasma, there are other factors to affect platelet function after TLE treatment. Exogenous fibrinogen did not completely restore platelet aggregation of normal platelets suspended in defibrinogenated plasma. Since PGI_2 was an important physiological inhibitor of platelet function *in vivo*, we measured the 6-keto $PGF_{1\alpha}$ level of plasmas during TLE infusion. Plasma 6-keto $PGF_{1\alpha}$ was significantly increased at 6-hour after TLE infusion (1.0 U/kg). Ancrod treatment in patients of glomerulonephritis could normalize platelet hyperaggregation *in vitro*,[45] it also restored PGI_2 generation capacity in patients with lupus nephritis with glomerular thrombi.[46] If this elevated PGI_2 was partially responsible for the reduced release reaction require further investigation. However, this elevated PGI_2 level is another advantage of using TLE in the treatment of patients with platelet hyperaggregability. Previous studies showed that plasmin exhibited either platelet activation or inhibition in a dose-dependent manner.[47-51] Nevertheless, in the present study the addition of aprotinin to the defibrinogenated plasma prior to suspending the normal washed platelets had no significant effect on platelet aggregation or ATP release. However, the elevation of FDPs at initial stage indicated the activation of endogenous fibrinolytic system. Whether plasmin caused the impairment of platelet function by a direct proteolytic effect on platelet membrane *in vivo* remained to be unclear.

Recent studies confirmed the relationships of blood viscosity to atherosclerosis, thrombosis and ischaemia.[52] However, it needs further investigation to clarify the role of blood viscosity on platelet function in long term basis although TLE indeed causes a significantly reduced blood viscosity.

We concluded that the long-lasting depleted plasma fibrinogen level is the primary factor responsible for the impaired platelet function in rabbits receiving TLE infusion. However, the brief elevation of FDPs at the early phase may partially be involved only during this stage. The elevated PGI_2 level at the later phase and other unknown factor(s) may be partially responsible for the impairment of platelet function (including release reaction). The reduced blood viscosity may also be beneficial to thrombo-embolic patients. Therefore, TLE therapy may be considered to be helpful in patients not only with venous thrombosis but also with arterial thrombotic disorders.

Acknowledgements

This work was supported by a grant from National Science Council to Taiwan (NSC82-0418-B0020097-BC).

REFEREMCES

1. Mahir MS, Hynd JW, Flute PT, and Dormandy JA (1987) Br J Surg 74: 508-510

2. Ewart MR, Hatton MWC, Basford JM, Dodgson KS (1970) Biochem J 118: 603-609

3. Turpie AGG, Prentice CRM, Mcnicol GP, Douglas AS (1971) Br J Haematol 20: 217-224

4. Rogoeczi E, Gergely J, Mcfarlane AS (1966) J Clin Invest 45: 1202-1212

5. Silberman S, Bernik MB, Potter EV, and Kwaan HC (1973) Br J Haematol 24: 101-113

6. Bell WR, Pitney WR, and Goodwin JF (1968) Lancet i: 490-493

7. Sharp AA, Warren BA, Paxton AM, and Allington MJ (1968) Lancet i: 493-499

8. Olsen EGJ, Pitney WR (1969) Br J Haematol 17: 425-429

9. Dormandy JA, Goyle KB, Reid HL (1977) Lancet i: 625-626

10. Lowe GDO, Campbell AF, Meek DR, Forbes CD, Prentice CRM (1978) Lancet ii: 698-700

11. Berglin E, Hansson HA, Teger-Nilsson AC, William-Olsson G (1976) Thromb Res 9: 81-93

12. Olsson P, Ljungqvist A, Goransson L (1973) Thromb Res 3: 161-172

13. Postlethwaite JC, Goyle KB, Dormandy JA, Hynd JW (1977) Br J Surg 64: 28-30

14. Latallo ZS (1983) Thromb Haemost 50: 604-609

15. Esnouf MP, Tunnah GW (1967) Br J Haematol 13: 581-590

16. Bell WR, Bolton G, Pitney WR (1968) Br J Haematol 15: 589-602

17. Brown CH, Bell WR, Shreiner DP, and Jackson DP (1972) J Lab Clin Med 79: 758-769

18. Slade CL, Andes WA, and Mason AD (1976) Thromb Haemost (Stuttg.) 36: 424-429

19. Prentice CRM, Hassanein AA, Turpe AGG, Mcnicol GP, Douglas AS (1969) Lancet i: 644-647

20. Martin DL, Hollinger RE, Suwanwela N, and Fedor EJ (1971) Fed Proc 30: 424 (abstr)

21. Seegers WH (1962) Prothrombin. 1962; Harvard University Press, Cambridge.

22. Warrell DA, Davidson NMcD, Greenwood BM, Ormerod LD, Pope HM, Watkins BJ, Prentice CRM (1977) Quart J Med 46: 33-62

23. Clauss VA (1957) Acta Haemat 17: 237-246

24. O'Brien JR (1962) J Clin Pathol 15: 452-455

25. DeLuca M and McElory WD (1978) Methods Enzymol 57: 3-15

26. Teng CM, Chen WY, Ko WC, Ouyang C (1987) Biochim Biophys Acta 924: 375-382

27. Orchard MA, Robinson C (1981) Br J Pharmacol 74: 206p

28. Blomback M, Egberg N, Johansson S-A, Johnsson H, Nillson SEG, and Blomback B (1971) Thromb Diath Haemorrh 45 (Suppl.): 51-61

29. Egberg N, Blomback M, Johnsson H, Abildgaard U, Blomback B, Diener G, Ekestrom S, Goransson L, Johansson S-A, McDonagh J, McDonagh R, Nilsson SE, Nordstrom S, Olsson P, and Wilman B (1971) Thromb Diath Haemorrh 47 (Suppl.): 379-387

30. Kowalski E, Kopec' M, and Wegrzyhowicz Z (1963) Thromb Diath Haemorrh (Stuttg) 10: 406-423

31. Jerushalmy Z, and Zucker MB (1965) Thromb Diath Haemorrh (Stuttg) 15: 413-419.

32. Tomikawa M, Iwamoto M, Soderman S, and Blomback B (1980) Thromb Res 19: 841-855

33. Kloczewiak M, Timmons S, and Hawiger J (1982) Biochem Biophys Res Commun 107: 181-187

34. Thorsen LI, Gogstad BG, Sletten K, and Solum NO (1986) Thromb Res 44: 611-623

35. Pasqua JJ, and Pizzo SV (1983) Biochim Biophy Acta 757: 282-287

36. Chen SC, Chou SH, and Thiagarajan P (1988) Biochemistry 27: 6121-6126

37. Kwaan HC, Barlow GH (1971) Thromb Diath Haemorrh (Suppl) 47: 361-369

38. Egberg N (1973) Acta Med Scand 194: 291-302

39. Gouin I, Lecompte T, Morel MC, Lebrazi J, Modderman PW, Kaplan C, and Samama MM (1992) Circulation 85: 935-941

40. Cross MJ (1964) Thromb Diath Haemorrh 12: 524-527

41. Inceman S, Caen J, Bernard J (1966) J Lab Clin Med 68: 21-32

42. Weiss HJ, and Rogers J (1971) N Engl J Med 285: 369-374

43. Meade TW, Vickers MV, Thompson SG, Stirling Y, Haines AP, Miller GJ (1985) Br Med J 290: 428-432

44. Huang TF, Sheu JR, Teng CM (1991) Thromb Haemost 66: 489-493

45. Pollak VE, Glueck HI, Weiss MA, Lebron-Berges A, and Miller MA (1982) Am J Nephrol 2: 195-207

46. Kant KS, Dosekun AK, Chandran KGP, Glas-Greenwalt P, Weiss MA, and Pollak VE (1982) Thromb Res 27: 651-658

47. Adelman B, Michelson AD, Loscalzo J, Greenberg J, and Handin RI (1985) Blood 65: 32-40

48. Guccione MA, Kinlough-Rathbone RL, Packman MA, Harfenist EJ, Rand ML, Greenberg JP, Perry DW, Harfenist EJ, Rand ML, Greenberg JP, Perry DW, Mustard JF (1985) Thromb Haemost 53: 8-14

49. Schafer AI, Adelman B (1985) J Clin Invest 75: 456-461

50. Schafer AI, Maas AK, Ware JA, Johnson PC, Rittenhous SE, Salzman EW (1986) J Clin Invest 78: 73-79

51. Coller BS (1990) N Engl J Med 322: 33-42

52. Lowe GDO (1992) Thromb Haemost 67: 494-498

Table 1. Plasma fibrinogen level, whole blood clotting time and whole blood
viscosity measured prior to and after the intravenous infusion of
thrombin-like enzyme (TLE) in rabbits.

	Control	TLE	
	0 h	6 h	24 h
Plasma fibrinogen (mg/dl)	239.7±8.2	33.9±7.5**	231.8±15.2
Whole blood clotting time (min)	4.1±0.2	IC$^+$,**	4.4±0.5
Whole blood viscosity (centipoise) At shear rate			
1.15 s^{-1}	14.69±1.09	8.68±0.54**	14.7±2.18
2.30 s^{-1}	9.34±0.54	5.68±0.27**	9.01±1.24
23.0 s^{-1}	4.54±0.22	3.34±0.18**	3.70±0.21*

These values are expressed as mean±SEM (n=6). The significant difference
between control (prior to) and 6 hrs and 24 hrs after TLE infusion were
expressed as *: P < 0.05; **: P < 0.001.
$^+$IC: Incoagulable (> 60 min).

EFFECT OF PLASMINOGEN ACTIVATOR ON PLATELET AGGREGATION

Akira SUEHIRO, Satoshi HIGASA, Motoo UEDA, Yoshio OURA, Yasuharu Nishida and Eizo KAKISHITA

2nd Department of Internal Medicine, Hyogo College of Medicine, 1-1 Mukogawa-cho, Nishinomiya, Hyogo, 663 JAPAN

KEY WORDS: Tissue-type plasminogen activator, Staphylokinase, Platelet aggregation.

ABSTRACT

The clinical efficacy of thrombolytic therapy with plasminogen activator (PA) may be partly influenced by its effect on blood platelets. We investigated the effect of PA on human platelet aggregation using as PAs, staphylokinase (SAK), which has been found to have higher specific thrombolytic properties and less fibrinogenolytic properties than those of streptokinase, and also recombinant tissue-type plasminogen activator (TPA). Platelet aggregation was evaluated using platelet-rich plasma (PRP) or washed platelet suspension (WP). To examine the effects of PA, platelets were preincubated with PA (final concentration range: 0.001–100 μ g/ml) at 37℃ for 30 minutes. Both TPA and SAK inhibited platelet aggregation induced by collagen and ADP in PRP only at high concentrations (50–100 μg/ml). Both agents did not inhibit PRP aggregation induced by ristocetin. Although TPA and SAK did not inhibit platelet aggregation induced by collagen in WP which contained 0.5 mM calcium and 25 mg/dl fibrinogen, both agents inhibited aggregation under the same conditions in WP when the platelets had been preincubated with these agents and plasminogen (0.5 U/ml). The most effective concentrations were 100 μg/ml for TPA and 1 μg/ml for SAK. These effects were inhibited by adding aprotinin (1000 U/ml). We concluded from these results that, PA can inhibit platelet aggregation in WP by generating of plasmin and/or fibrinogen degradation products, but is only partially effective in PRP, possibly because of the existence of plasmin inhibitor.

INTRODUCTION

Although the clinical usefulness of thrombolytic therapy for myocardial infarction, deep vein thrombosis, pulmonary embolism and other arterial thrombosis has been evaluated [1,2], several problems limit the effectiveness of thrombolytic agents, including failure of thrombolysis, reocclusion after thrombolysis and also hemorrhage complications [3]. These problems may be partly related to the effect of thrombolytic agents on platelet function [4]. Previous in vitro studies have shown that plasminogen activator (PA) may induce both inhibition [5,6,7] and activation [7,8,9] of platelet functions.

In this study, we investigated the effect of PA on human platelet aggregation using staphylokinase (SAK), which has been found to have higher specific thrombolytic properties and less fibrinogenolytic properties than those of streptokinase [10,11], in comparison with re-combinant tissue-type plasminogen activator (TPA), a typical PA.

MATERIALS AND METHODS

Chemicals

SAK (1 mg/ml) solution in 10 mM phosphate buffer (pH 6.8) was supplied by Yakult Central Institute, Tokyo. TPA (Genentech) was purchased from Kyowa Hakko Kogyo, Tokyo, and aprotinin (Behringwerke) was from Hoechst Japan, Tokyo. Plasminogen from human plasma was from Sigma Chemical, St. Louis.

Platelet preparation

Human platelets were obtained from healthy donors who had taken no medication for at least 10 days. Venous blood was drawn into 3.8% sodium citrate (1:9 v/v). Platelet-rich plasma (PRP) and platelet-poor plasma (PPP) were obtained by centrifugation of the citrated blood at room temperature for 10 minutes at 150 x g and for 15 minutes at 3,000 x g, respec-tively. Platelet count in PRP was adjusted with PPP to 200,000/μl. To obtain a washed plate-let suspension (WP), platelets in PRP were washed twice with Tyrode solutin buffered by 10 mM HEPES with 1 mM EDTA and resuspended in Tyrode solution buffered by 10 mM HEPES, and the platelet count was adjusted to 200,000/μl.

Platelet aggregation

Platelet aggregation after adenosine diphosphate (ADP, Sigma Chemical Co.), collagen (Hormon-Chemie) and ristocetin (Sigma Chemical Co.) was monitored at 37℃ with stirring using an aggregometer (Hema Tracer, NBS). To examine the effects of TPA and SAK on platelet aggregation, PRP or WP was preincubated with these agents (final concentration range: 0.001-100 μg/ml) at 37℃ for 30 minutes without stirring.

RESULTS

Both TPA (Fig. 1 A and B) and SAK (Fig. 2 A and B) significantly inhibited platelet aggrega-tion in PRP induced by ADP (2 μM) and collagen (2 μg/ml) at high concentrations (50-100 μg/ml), but not at low concentrations of less than 50 μg/ml. Both agents did not inhibit platelet aggregation in PRP induced by ristocetin (1.5 mg/ml) even at 100 μg/ml (Fig. 1 C, Fig. 2 C). When WP was preincubated with TPA or SAK together with 0.5 mM calcium and 25 mg/dl fibrinogen at 37℃ for 30 minutes, collagen (10 μg/ml)-induced aggregation was significantly inhibited only at 100 μg/ml TPA (Fig. 3, 4). When plasminogen (0.5 U/ml) was added to the preincubation fluid, both TPA and SAK inhibited platelet aggregation even at relatively low concentrations (Fig. 3, 4). The most effective concentrations were 100 μg/ml for TPA and 1 μg/ml for SAK. The inhibitory effects of TPA (10 μg/ml) and SAK (1 μg/ml) recovered to the control level on addition of aprotinin (1000 U/ml) (Fig. 5). However, this effect of aprotinin on the inhibition of TPA (100 μg/ml) was only a partial one (Fig. 5).

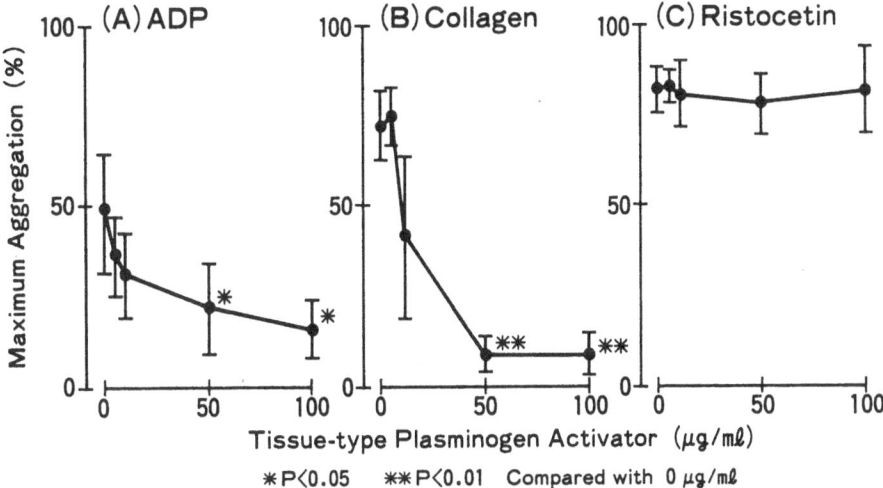

Fig. 1 Effect of TPA on platelet aggregation in PRP induced by (A) ADP (2 μ M), (B) collagen (2 μg/ml), or (C) ristocetin (1.5 mg/ml). Each value represents the mean $\pm$ S.D. of 5 experiments.

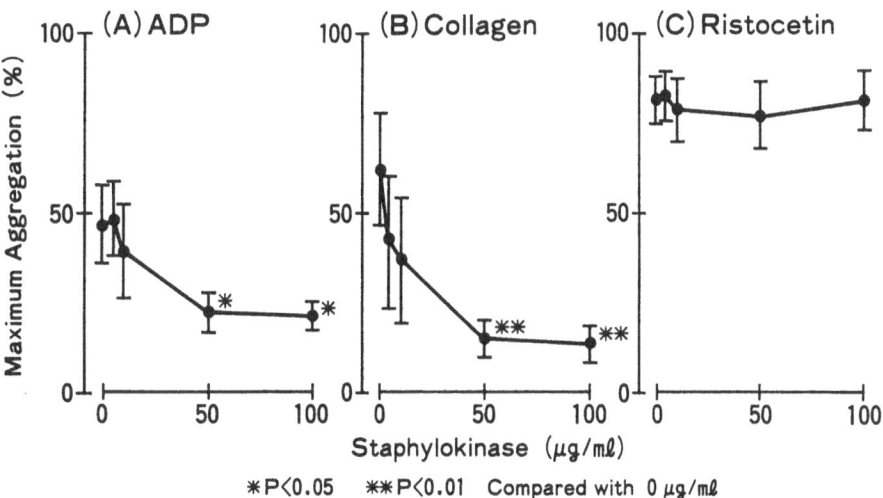

Fig. 2 Effect of SAK on platelet aggregation in PRP induced by (A) ADP (2 μ M), (B) collagen (2 μg/ml), or (C) ristocetin (1.5 mg/ml). Each value represents the mean $\pm$ S.D. of 5 experiments.

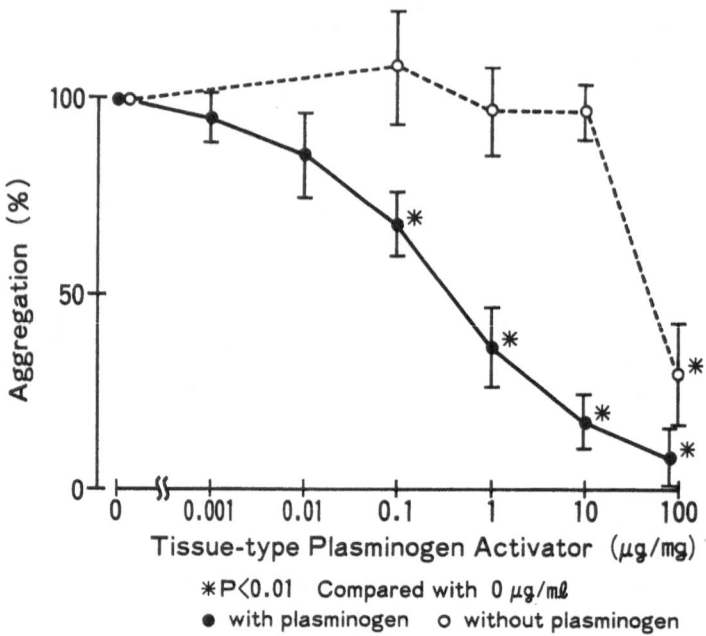

Fig. 3 Effect of TPA on collagen (10 μg/ml)–induced platelet aggregation in WP. Each value represents the mean ± S.D. of 4–6 experiments.

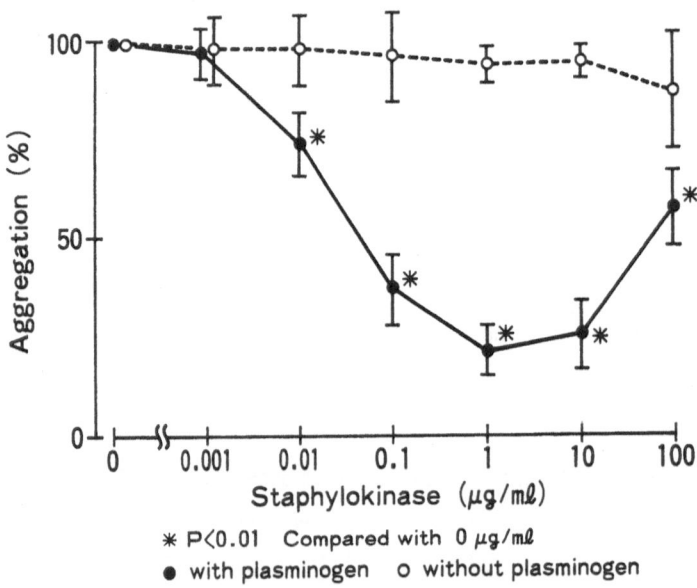

Fig. 4 Effect of SAK on collagen (10 μg/ml)–induced platelet aggregation in WP. Each value represents the mean ± S.D. of 4–5 experiments.

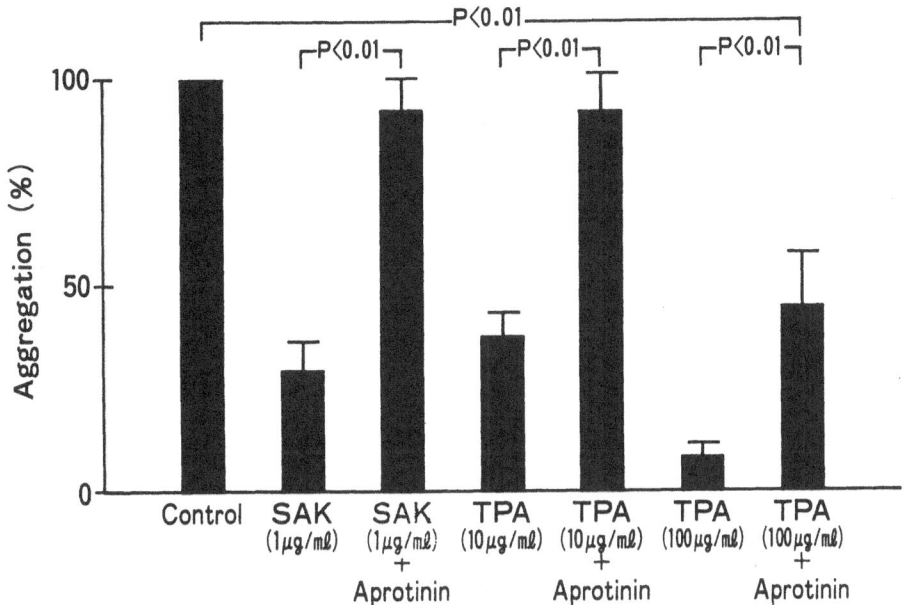

Fig. 5 Effect of aprotinin on inhibition of collagen (10 μ g/ml)–induced platelet aggregation by PA in WP. Each value represents the mean ± S.D. of 3–5 experiments.

DISCUSSION

The effect of PA on platelet function in vitro is complicated as there is evidence of both platelet inhibition [5,6,7] and activation [7,8,9]. Although most studies have shown that the PA effect results in plasmin or fibrinogen degradation products generated in an in vitro reaction system, a direct effect of PA on platelets has also been suggested [12]. In this study, we chose SAK, which dose not have enzymatic activity itself and acts as a plasminogen activator only when it forms a complex with plasminogen, which has high specific thrombolytic proper-ties [10,11], to examine the effect on platelet aggregation in comparison with TPA.

As both TPA and SAK inhibited platelet aggregation in WP only when platelets were pre-incubated with plasminogen, these PAs seem to affect platelets by generating plasmin and/or fibrinogen degradation prodults in the reaction fluid. This hypothesis was further supported by the result that aprotinin, an inhibitor of plasmin, inhibited the effect of TPA and SAK. Only the highest concentration of TPA (100 μ g/ml) inhibited platelet aggregation in WP even under the condition without plasminogen. However, this effect is thought to be non–specific due to contamination by L–arginine in commercially available TPA from Genentech. Evidence for this comes from the result that aprotinin only partially, and not com-pletely, inhibited the effect of 100 μ g/ml TPA. A recent paper also reports that L–arginine itself inhibits the increase of cytoplasmic calcium, suggesting platelet inhibition as observed with TPA [7].

In PRP, both TPA and SAK did not inhibit platelet aggregation except at relatively high concentrations of more than 50 μ g/ml. This result suggests that PA is not as effective on platelets in the human body, although PA itself has an inhibitory effect under experimental conditions without plasma components. The existence of alpha-2 anti-plasmin in PRP may restrict the effect of PA [13], although the detailed mechanism remains to be clarified.

We cannot yet clarify the mechanism of platelet inhibition by PA or plasmin, but our findings that TPA and SAK inhibited platelet aggregation induced by ADP and collagen, which aggregate platelets through glycoprotein (GP) IIb–IIIa in platelet membrane, and did not inhibit that induced by ristocetin, which aggregates platelets through GP Ib, suggest that PA or its products affect platelets through GPIIb–IIIa but not GPIb. A recent study indicates that plasmin changes the migration of GPIIb–IIIa judging from autoradiograms of SDS–PAGE gels [5], which offers support for our hypothesis.

In conclusion, PA inhibited platelet aggregation in WP by the generation of plasmin and/or fibrinogen degradation products, whereas the inhibitory effects were only partial in PRP possibly because of the existence of alpha-2 anti-plasmin.

REFERENCES

1. Haber, E., Quertermous, T., Matsueda, G.R. and Runge, M.S. (1989) Sience 243, 51–56.
2. Collen, D., Stamp, D.C. and Gold, H.K. (1988) Ann.Rev.Med. 39, 405–423.
3. Coller, B.S. (1990) N.Engl.J.Med. 322,33–42.
4. Bertolino, G., Noris, P., Previtali, M., Gamba, G., Ferrario, M., Montani, N. and Bolduini, C.L. (1992) Am.J.Cardiol. 69, 457–461.
5. Torr, S.R., Winters, K.J., Santoro, S.A. and Sobel, B.E. (1990) Thromb.Res. 59, · 279–293.
6. Fears, R., Ferres, H. and Greenwood, H.C. (1990) Thromb.Res. 60, 259–265.
7. Penny, W.F., Ware, J.A. (1992) Blood 79, 91–98.
8. Yamada, Y., Furui, H., Furumichi, T., Yamauchi, K., Yokota, M. and Saito, H. (1990) Am.Heart J. 121, 1618–1627.
9. Vaugham, D.E., Houtte, E.V., Declerck, P.J., Collen, D. (1991) Circulation 84, 84–91.
10. Matsuo, O., Okada, K., Fukao, H., Tomioka, Y., Ueshima, S., Watanuki, M. and Sakai, M. (1990) Blood 76, 925–929.
11. Sakai, M., Watanuki, M. and Matsuo, O. (1989) Biochem.Biophys.Res.Comm. 162, 830–837.
12. Vaugham, D.E., Mendelsohn, M.E., Declerck, P.J., Houttle, E.V., Collen, D. and Loscalzo, J. (1989) J.Biol.Chem. 264, 15869–15874.
13. Wiman, B. (1980) Biochem.J. 191, 229–232.

ARACHIDONATE 12-LIPOXYGENASE OF HUMAN PLATELETS

Shozo Yamamoto, Satoshi Matsuda[+], Jun Murakami, Yasuchika Yamamoto, Yumiko Konishi[+], Chieko Yokoyama, Toshiya Arakawa, Yoshitaka Takahashi, Tanihiro Yoshimoto, Yasuo Mimura[+], and Minoru Okuma[++]

Departments of Biochemistry and [+]Ophthalmology, Tokushima University, School of Medicine, Tokushima 770, and [++]Department of Internal Medicine, Kyoto University, Faculty of Medicine, Kyoto 606, Japan

Thromboxane A_2 is well known as a proaggregatory and vasoconstrictive compound [1]. It is produced from arachidonic acid in platelets, and fatty acid cyclooxygenase responsible for the thromboxane synthesis is localized in the microsomal fraction of human platelets [2]. There is another metabolic pathway of arachidonic acid in human platelets. The pathway is initiated by the reaction of arachidonate 12-lipoxygenase, which is localized predominantly in the cytosol of human platelets [3].

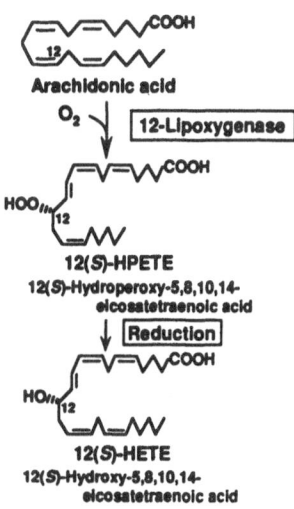

Fig. 1 Arachidonate 12-lipoxygenase.

As shown in Fig. 1, 12-lipoxygenase oxygenates the position-12 of arachidonic acid counted starting from the carboxyl carbon. The primary product is 12S-hydroperoxy-5,8,10,14-eicosatetraenoic acid, which is usually referred to as 12-HPETE. In a whole cell preparation or a crude enzyme preparation the 12-hydroperoxide is reduced either enzymatically or non-enzymatically to 12S-hydroxy-5,8,10,14-eicosatetraenoic acid, which is abbreviated as 12-HETE. Since 12-lipoxygenase was found in human platelets as the first mammalian lipoxygenase in 1974 [4], the enzyme has been found not only in platelets but also in leukocytes and various other tissues of several animal species [5-8]. In contrast to cyclooxygenase and 5-lipoxygenase, which synthesize bioactive prostaglandins, thromboxanes and leukotrienes, any enzymatic product with a specific biological activity and an established stereochemical structure has not yet been found in the metabolic pathway initiated by the 12-lipoxygenase, and the enzyme has been ignored by most investigators until recently.

Our biochemical, immunological and molecular biological studies in the last decade have demonstrated that there are two isoforms of 12-lipoxygenase. They are distinguishable each other in terms of substrate specificity and immunogenicity. Leukocyte 12-lipoxygenases have a broad substrate specificity, and they are active not only with arachidonic acid and other C_{20} fatty acids but also with C_{18} fatty acids like linoleic and linolenic acids [8,9]. In contrast, platelet 12-lipoxygenases are almost inactive with linoleic and linolenic acids [9,10]. Furthermore, no cross-reactivity is found between the antibodies raised against the leukocyte and platelet enzymes [9], and a relatively low identity of amino acid sequences was observed between two types of 12-lipoxygenase [11]. The leukocyte-type enzyme was found not only in leukocytes but also in parenchymal cells of human adrenal [12], bovine trachea [13], porcine pituitary [14] and canine brain [15]. The platelet-type enzyme has so far been found only in platelets of several animal species.

As I mentioned above, a general theory of 12-lipoxygenase physiology has not been established. However, various findings of physiological interest have been reported. First, Murota and others reported that a low concentration of 12-HETE stimulated vascular smooth muscle cell migration. 5-HETE or 15-HETE was much less active. Secondly, according to Schwartz and others, certain 12-lipoxygenase metabolites are the second messengers in the neurotransmission of Aplysia ganglion. Involvement of hepoxilin A3 in rat hippocampal neurotransmission was reported by Pace-Asciak and others. The hepoxilin is so far known as a non-enzymatic degradation product of 12-HPETE. Thirdly, Pace-Asciak's group reported that hepoxilin A3 is also a stimulator of insulin secretion. Furthermore, according to Honn and associates 12-HETE may express or activate the GPIIb/IIIa-like receptor which is involved in the metastasis of tumor cells. Dray and his coworkers reported that the 12-lipoxygenase products are also involved in the secretion of LH-RH by hypothalamus and of melatonin by pineal gland. Nadler's group proposed an essential role of 12-lipoxygenase metabolite in the angiotensin-dependent secretion of aldosterone. All these findings (See the original papers cited in reference 7) are really interesting, but further investigations are required for a general story applicable to many animal tissues and species.

In 1979 Okuma and Uchino investigated the patients with myeloproliferative disorders such as polycythemia vera, chronic myeloid leukemia, essential thrombocythemia and myelofibrosis, and found that 18 out of 33 patients showed a decreased 12-lipoxygenase activity of platelets [16]. Later Schafer also reported a reduced 12-lipoxygenase activity in 24 out of 60 patients [17]. On the basis of our recent molecular biological studies on 12-lipoxygenases, we reinvestigated this finding. As presented in Fig. 2, when the platelet cytosol fraction was incubated with radioactive arachidonic acid and the products were separated by thin layer chromatography, the enzyme of a normal subject gave radioactive peaks of 12-HPETE and 12-HETE. We tested two patients with polycythemia vera and a patient with essential thrombocythemia, but almost no arachidonate oxygenation was observed in platelets of the three patients [18].

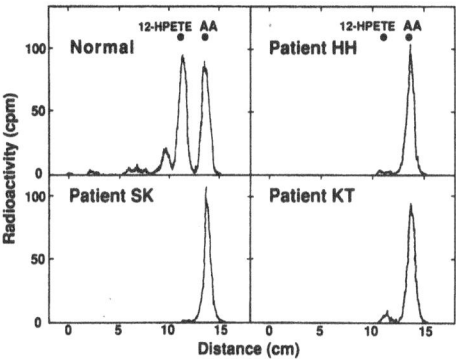

Fig. 2 Deficiency of 12-lipoxygenase activity in platelets of three patients with myeloproliferative disorders.

Previously we prepared monoclonal antibodies against the human platelet 12-lipoxygenase for the purpose of immunoaffinity purification of this somewhat unstable enzyme. A crude enzyme was given to mice as an antigen, and two clones producing anti-12-lipoxygenase antibody were isolated by the hybridoma technique [18]. The two antibodies are known to recognize different sites of the 12-lipoxygenase protein. These antibodies cross-reacted with bovine platelet-12-lipoxygenase, but not with porcine and bovine leukocyte 12-lipoxygenases [9]. By the use of the two monoclonal anti-12-lipoxygenase antibodies, we set up a peroxidase-linked immunoassay of sandwich-type for quantitative determination of 12-lipoxygenase protein. In routine assays 96-well plastic plates are used, and the surface of each well is coated with one of the two anti-lipoxygenase antibodies, to which the 12-lipoxygenase protein is bound. According to the biotin-avidin method, the other antibody is biotinylated, and incubated with the immobilized 12-lipoxygenase protein. The immunocomplex is then bound to an avidin-peroxidase conjugate. The amount of 12-lipoxygenase protein is determined by the assay of the peroxidase activity of the immobilized immunocomplex. The human platelet 12-lipoxygenase has not been purified to homogeneity, and we can not use a purified enzyme as a standard. Therefore, the amount of 12-lipoxygenase protein is expressed as the increase of absorbance at 492 nm due to the peroxidase product. The peroxidase activity increased in a linear fashion as the amount of the platelet cytosol was raised. The peroxidase-linked immunoassay is about 20-fold more sensitive than the 12-lipoxygenase activity assay with radioactive arachidonic acid as substrate. As shown in Fig. 3, the platelet cytosol fractions of the three patients with much lower levels of 12-lipoxygenase activity were subjected to the peroxidase-linked immunoassay. As compared with the average value of 8 normal subjects, the three patients showed negligible levels of 12-lipoxygenase protein in their platelets.

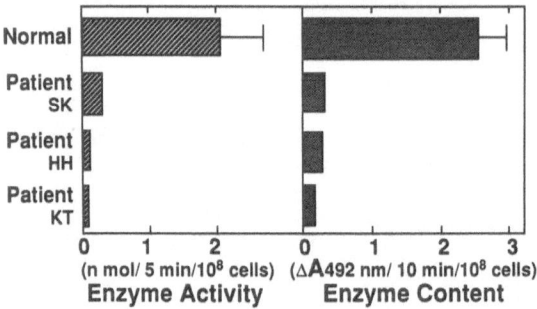

Fig. 3 Decreased 12-lipoxygenase protein and activity in platelets of three patients with myeloproliferative disorders.

Furthermore, we determined the level of 12-lipoxygenase mRNA in the platelets of the patients [18]. Since there is little amount of mRNA in human platelet cells, we carried out a sensitive polymerase chain reaction with an internal standard cRNA, which was prepared by a 105-bp deletion of a 12-lipoxygenase cDNA clone [11]. Total RNA of human platelets and the internal standard cRNA were mixed, reverse-transcribed, and the single-strand cDNAs were subjected to PCR amplification with 5'- and 3'-primers specific for the human platelet 12-lipoxygenase. A linear relationship was observed between the platelet number and the amount of 12-lipoxygenase mRNA, which was determined by the radioactivity of incorporated dCMP and then calculated with reference to the internal standard.

As shown in Fig. 4, a normal subject and a patient with essential thrombocythemia were examined by the standard PCR method. With reference to the 361-bp bands derived from the internal standard cRNA, we compared the density of amplified 12-lipoxygenase cDNA fragments with a size of 466 bp. The patient showed a much lower density than the normal subject. The average of 12-lipoxygenase mRNA content was about 4.7 ng/10^{11} platelets as determined with 13 normal subjects. All the three patients showed much lower mRNA levels (0.15, 0.11 and 0.10 ng/10^{11} cells). Thus,

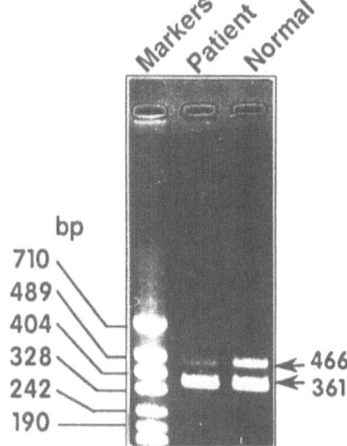

Fig. 4 PCR amplification of 12-lipoxygenase mRNA in a normal subject and a patient with myeloproliferative disorder.

the decreased 12-lipoxygenase activity in platelets of the three patients with myeloproliferative disorders could be attributed to the decrease in mRNA and protein of 12-lipoxygenase. The molecular mechanism underlying such an impaired expression of the 12-lipoxygenase gene awaits further analysis of the patients' gene and transcription factors.

References

[1] Hamberg M, Svensson J, Samuelsson B (1975) Proc Natl Acad Sci USA 72: 2994-2998

[2] Hammarström S, Falardeau P (1977) Proc Natl Acad Sci USA 74: 3691-3695

[3] Siegel MI, McConnell RT, Porter NA, Cuatrecasas P (1980) Proc Natl Acad Sci USA 77: 308-312

[4] Hamberg M, Samuelsson B (1974) Proc Natl Acad Sci USA 71: 3400-3404

[5] Nugteren DH (1975) Biochim Biophys Acta 380: 299-307

[6] Yamamoto S (1991) Free Radical Biology and Medicine 10: 149-159

[7] Yamamoto S (1992) Biochim Biophys Acta in press

[8] Yokoyama C, Shinjo F, Yoshimoto T, Yamamoto S, Oates JA, Brash AR (1986) J Biol Chem 261: 16714-16721

[9] Takahashi Y, Ueda N, Yamamoto S (1988) Arch Biochem Biophys 266: 613-621

[10] Hada T, Ueda N, Takahashi Y, Yamamoto S. (1991) Biochim Biophys Acta 1083: 89-93

[11] Yoshimoto T, Yamamoto Y, Arakawa T, Suzuki H, Yamamoto S, Yokoyama C. Tanabe T, Toh H (1990) Biochem Biophys Res Commun 172: 1230-1235

[12] Nadler JL, Gu J-L, Rossi J, Yoshimoto T, Yamamoto S, Natarajan R (1992) The 8th International Conference on Prostaglandins and Related Compounds, Abstracts p.165

[13] Hansbrough JR, Takahashi Y, Ueda N, Yamamoto S, Holtzman, MJ (1990) J Biol Chem 265: 1771-1776

[14] Ueda N, Kaneko S, Yoshimoto T, Yamamoto S (1986) J Biol Chem 261: 7982-7988

[15] Nishiyama M, Okamoto H, Watanabe T, Hori T, Hada T, Ueda N, Yamamoto S, Tsukamoto H, Watanabe K, Kirino T (1992) J Neurochem 58: 1395-1400

[16] Okuma M, Uchino H (1979) Blood 54: 1258-1271

[17] Schafer AI (1982) N Engl J Med 306: 381-386

[18] Matsuda S, Murakami J, Yamamoto Y, Konishi Y, Yokoyama C, Yoshimoto T, Yamamoto S, Mimura Y, Okuma M (1992) Biochim Biophys Acta in press

CLINICAL EFFECT OF ANTIPLATELET THERAPY FOR CEREBRAL THROMBOSIS
- COMPARISON OF TWO GROUPS WITH DIFFERENT CONTROL OF HYPERAGGREGABILITY -

Y. HOMMA,[1] A. HATTORI,[2] S. ITO,[3] Niigata stroke and antiplatelet therapy study group
[1] Neurology department, Sado general hospital, Chigusa, Kanai, Sadogun, Niigataken, Japan 952-12
[2] Niigata University of medicine
[3] Niigata South hospital

Keyword : low dose aspirin and ticlopidine therapy

INTRODUCTION

Increased platelet function, such as hyperaggregability, is one of the risk factors of cerebral infarction, like hypertension and diabetes. Control of platelet aggregability with antiplatelet drugs is significant therepeutic treatment for the prevention of cerebral infarction. Aspirin and ticlopidine, both of which are irreversible antiplatelet drugs, have established efficacy in the prevention of second cerebral thrombosis [1] [2]. However, their clinical application, that is how to use aspirin and ticlopidine, have not been clarified in sufficient detail. In 1991 Uchiyama et al [3] demonstrated that the combination therapy of low doses of aspirin and ticlopidine suppressed the multiple pathways involved in platelet aggregation. We have studied this combination therapy using the flexible dose methoed for 8 years for the prevention of second cerebral thrombosis with individualized therapeutic goals [4]. During this period, we tried to find answers to the following questions.

1. To which level should hyperaggregability be controlled ?

2. Is control to normoaggregability sufficient for the prevention of cerebral thrombosis ?

3. How frequent are hemorrhagic accidents in association with antiplatelet therapy ?

SUBJECTS AND METHODS

In this prospective study, 173 patients with cerebral thrombosis who had hyperaggregability received flexible-dose therapy with a low dose of aspirin and/or ticlopidine. Three quarters of the patients had lacunar infarction and the remaining had atherothrombosis of the main trunk or cortical branches. The patients were divided into two groups. One group had a therapeutic goal of normal aggregability and was referred to as the normalized group. The other group had a therapeutic goal of maintenance of hypoaggregability and was referred to as the lowered group.

The platelet aggregation test was performed with a standard aggregometer using two concentrations of aggregants, ADP and collagen respectivey.(Table 1)

Table 1. Platelet aggregation test using turbidometry

Agonist	high conc.	low conc.
ADP	10 μM	1.0 μM
Collagen	2.0 μg/mℓ	0.5 μg/mℓ

platelet rich plasma (plt. conc. 300×10^9/L)

Many parameters have been proposed for the assessment of aggregability. In this study, the maximum aggregation rate was used. The normal range was set as follows : the maximum rate of aggregation induced by the high concentration of aggregants were more than 50 %, and that induced by the low concentration of aggregants were less than 50 %.

An evaluation of hyperaggregability was made when the maximum rate of aggregation induced by a low concentration of aggregants was more than 50 %. An evaluation of hypoaggregability was made when the maximum rate of aggregation induced by a high concentration of aggregants was less than 50 %. Suppression of the maximum aggregation rate to below 20 % was avoided because such treatment was known to be associated with the heightened risk of bleeding.

Table 2. The patient characteristics of the two groups

	normalized group	lowerd group	
No. of patients	130	43	
(male : female)	(74 : 56)	(25 : 18)	N.S
age (years)	$70 \pm 10.6^{*}$	69 ± 14.1	
duration of treatment (months)	30.9 ± 25.5	27.8 ± 27.2	N.S
other risk factors	Hypertension		$p < 0.05$
	Diabetes and Hyperlipidemia		N.S

$*$: mean $\pm$ SD

The patient characteristics of the two groups are shown in Table 2. For both groups the mean age was about 70 years and the mean duration of treatment was about 30 months. There were no significant differences between the two groups. Among other risk factors hypertension was more frequent among patients in the normalized group than in the lowered group. The reasons for the 3 times greater sample size in the normalized group are as follows. The major reason was that the attending physicians hesitated to expose patients to lowered aggregability for fear of hemorrhagic accidents. Therefore, the therapeutic goal was deliberately set at normal aggregability in those patients with peptic ulcers, hemorrhoid, uncontrollable hypertension or unruptured cerebral aneurysm, or a history of cancer, or who were predisposed to petechiae or epistaxis.

Table 3. Antiplatelet drugs used in this study

— antiplatelet drug —

Aspirin	$10 \sim 81$ mg/day
Ticlopidine	$100 \sim 300$ mg/day

modified according to the patient's condition

The most frequent doses

	normalized group	lowered group
Aspirin	20 mg	30 mg
Ticlopidine	100 mg	200 mg

In this trial, aspirin and ticlopidine were administtted orally, modifing those doses according to the patient's condition.(Table 3) Other potent antiplatelet agents were not used.

RESULTS

The results of this trial are shown in Table 4. In the normalized group, 16 out of 130 patients experienced recurrence of completed strokes. The annual recurrence rate was caluculated as 4.9%. In the lowered group, recurrence was not observed in any of the 43 patients. This difference in the recurrence rate was statistically signifcant (Fisher's direct probability test).

Table 4. Result of antiplatelet therapy

| | platelet aggregability | |
	normalized group	lowered group
subjects	130 patients	43 patients
reccurence	16 patients	none
annual reccurence rate	4.9 %	0 %
hemorrhagic accidents	10 patients	4 patients
annual incidence of hemorrhagic accidents	3.0 %	4.1 %

Hemorrhagic accidents occurred at an incidence of 3.0% and 4.1% in the respective groups, but these valuses did not differ significantly (Table 5). The major accident was gastrointestinal bleeding and there were no cases of cerebral hemorrhage.

Table 5. Details of the hemorrhagic accidents

| | platelet aggregability | | |
	normalized group	lowered group	total
hematemesis	4	2	6 patients
melena	2	1	3 patients
hemorrhage from hemorrhoids (severe)	1 (died)	none	1 patients
nasal hemorrhage (severe)	2	none	2 patients
genital hemorrhage	none	1	1 patients
subcutaneous hemorrhage	1	none	1 patients
cerebral hemorrhage	none	none	none
total	10/130	4/43	14/173
annual incidence of hemorrhagic accidents	3.0 %	4.1 %	3.3 %

DISCUSION

The extent to which platelets are involved in the development of cerebral infarction depends on the pathological type of the condition [5]. Antiplatelet therapy should be performed in pathological types with increased platelet aggregability. Therefore, this trial was conducted in patients with lacunar infarction and atherothrombosis, those with cardiogenic embolism and low perfusion infarction were not enrolled in the trial.

To avoid the "aspirin dilemma", the dose of aspirin should be limited to 80 mg or less [6]. Furthermore, a lower dose of aspirin is safer because the drug has high gastrotoxicity [7]. Aspirin therapy was started at a dose of 10 mg/day, which was modified according to the collagen-induced aggregation within the range with a maximum of 81 mg/day. The dose of ticlopidine was adjusted to 100-300 mg/day while monitoring ADP-induced aggregation.

When should antiplatelet therapy be started ? Antiplatelet therapy should be started as soon as the patient enters a chronic condition since clinical practice has suggested that cerebral infarction likely to recur sooner after the first attack. Most of the subjects in this trial began to receive this therapy 8 weeks after the first attack.

Long-term treatment with the usual dose of aspirin leads to a reduction in its clinical benefit becauses of its gastrotoxicity [7] while treatment with 500 mg ticlopidine is usually associated with high incidence of adverse reactions including diarrhea and skin rash [6]. Antiplatelet therapy does not require such high doses. With respect to the levels of aggregation induced by ADP and collagen, the combination of a low dose of aspirin and 100-300 mg ticlopidine as used in this trial is thought sufficient. Fixed dose method is not appropriate for the treatment of individual patients and may have a high medicolegal risk even though efficacy can be attained in patients in general.

In antiplatelet therapy, the therapeutic doses should be tailored for individual patients taking account of its aggregability.

CONCLUSION

Now attempting the trial of antiplatelet therapy, it might not be allowed to set true placebo because the efficacy of antiplatelet therapy has been already confirmed.

Comparing the two groups of the patients adjusting to normalized aggregability and lowered one, we have clarified the efficacy to correct hyperaggregabily to hypoaggregability.

We would like to say that such a high dose of autiplatelet agents as that of past trials is not necessary. Antiplatelet therapy should be selected by taking account of the condition of platelet aggregability for indivisual patients.

REFERENCES

1) Gent M, Blakely J, Easton JD, Ellis DJ, Hachinski VC, Harrison JW, Panak E, Robert RS, Sicurella J, Turpie AGG, and The CATS group (1989) Lancet i : 1215-1220

2) Hass WK, Easton JD, Adams HP Jr, Pryse-Phillips W, Molony BA, Anderson S, Kamm B for the Ticlopidine Aspirin Stroke study Group (1989) N Engl J Med 321 : 501-507

3) Uchiyama S, Sone R, Nagayama T, Shibagaki Y, Kobayashi I, Maruyama S, Kusakabe K (1989) Stroke 20 : 1643-1647

4) Hattori A and SATS group (1990) Niigata medical J 104 : 381-386

5) Waki R, Okada Y, Tashiro M, Miyashita T, Yamaguchi T (1987) Jpn. J. Stroke 9 : 433-439

6) Hanley SP, Bevan J, Cockbill SR, Heptinstall S (1981) Lanset i : 969-971

7) The ESPS group (1987) Lancet i : 1351-1354

EFFECTS OF INTRACELLULAR pH ON THE ANTITHROMBOTIC PROPERTIES OF HUMAN VASCULAR ENDOTHELIAL CELLS

MASAHITO YAMAGAMI, SHOHEI SAWADA, TOSHIYUKI TAMAGAKI, KYOICHIRO KOBAYASHI, KAZUHARU KATO, KATSUMI YAMAMOTO, KAORU SHIRAI, KEIZO YAMADA, HARUCHIKA MASUDA, KATSUMI NAKAGAWA, HAJIME TSUJI AND MASAO NAKAGAWA.
Second Department of Medicine, Kyoto Prefectural University of Medicine, Kyoto, Japan

Introduction

Among the many events that occur in stimulated cells, there is always a significant shift in intracellular pH ([pH]i). The expression of some cellular responses after stimulation have been attributed to this pH shift. In neutrophils, stimulus-induced alkaline shifts in [pH]i have been proposed to modulate chemotaxis, aggregation, phagocytosis, secretion and the generation of superoxide radicals[1]-[3]. In recent years, a convincing role for changes in [pH]i in the action of extracellular growth stimulation has been documented with a variety of cell types in culture[4]. However, the relationship between [pH]i and the antithrombotic mechanisms of vascular endothelial cells has not been investigated. In the present study, the effects of [pH]i on the antithrombotic properties of vascular endothelial cells were investigated utilizing human umbilical vein endothelial cells (HUVEC).

MATERIALS AND METHODS

1) Culture of vascular endothelial cells

The culture of vascular endothelial cells was performed by the previously described method[5], and primary cultured cells that formed confluent monolayers were used in the following experiments.

The cells were identified as vascular endothelial cells by detecting Weibel-Palade bodies on electron microscopy, and the release of angiotensin I converting enzyme.

2) Measurement of cytosolic free Ca^{++} concentration

The cytosolic free Ca^{++} concentration was measured by the modified method of Grynkiewicz[6]. In short, the endothelial cells were scraped from the dishes with a rubber spatula and collected in centrifugation tubes. The cells were then rinsed with 10 ml of a conditioned buffer solution without Ca^{++} (buffer A without Ca^{++}: 150mM NaCl, 5mM KCl, 1mM $MgCl_2$, 5mM glucose, 10mM HEPES, pH 7.4) containing 1.0% bovine serum albumin. After the cells were resuspended in 3 ml of the solution, they were incubated with 3.2 μM fura-2/AM at 37 °C for 45 min and subsequently diluted to 20 ml with the solution. They were then centrifuged at 250G for 10 min, following resuspension in the 1.0 % bovine serum albumin solution (cell counts were 10^6/ml). Fluorescence signals from the endothelial cell suspensions were recorded in UV-compatible cuvettes utilizing a Ca^{++} analyzer CAF-100 (Japan Spectroscopic Co., LTD. Tokyo, Japan).

Key words: Prostacyclin; Cytosolic calcium; Intracellular pH
　　　　　　　Calcium storage site; Human vascular endothelial cell

3)Measurement of intracellular pH

[pH]i in HUVEC was determined using a pH sensitive dye, 2,7,bis-(carboxyethyl)-carboxyfluorescein-AM(BCECF-AM) as described by Rink et al[7]. The cells were harvested in HEPES buffer (153.0mM Nacl, 5.0mM KCl, 5.0mM glucose, 10.0mM HEPES pH 7.4) and incubated for 40 min at 37 °C with $3 \mu M$ BCECF-AM. The ratio of fluorescence intensity was determined with a Ca^{++} analyzer CAF-100 using an excitation wavelength of 450 and 500 nm, and an emission wavelength of 540 nm. At the end of the experiment, the signal was calibrated by lysing the cells with digitonin and measuring the ratio of fluorescence intensity at known pH values. To correct for the red shift in the spectrum of BCECF induced by calibrating BCECF after lysing cells with digitonin, intact cells were incubated in a high K^+ buffer, and known pH values were imposed inside the cells using $10 \mu g/ml$ nigericin. The cells were then lysed with digitonin, and a new calibration curve was constructed. The calibration curve was linear between the pH range 6.6-7.8, and correction was made as described by Thomas et al[8]. The changes in [pH]i observed after the addition of the test agents was determined from the point when the stimulator was added to the point when no further enhancement of [pH]i was observed. Using this measurement, the resting [pH]i in HUVEC was determined to be 7.17 ± 0.03.

4)Assay of prostacyclin concentration

HUVEC were incubated with $500 \mu l$ of buffer A (150mM NaCl, 5mM KCl, 1mM $MgCl_2$, 1.8mM $CaCl_2$, 5mM glucose, 10mM HEPES, pH 7.4) containing several test reagents in 37 °C for 15 min, and an aliquot was subjected to the assay of prostacyclin concentration. Prostaglandins mainly generated from HUVEC were confirmed to be prostacyclin by thin-layer chromatography from a preliminary experiment with $[1-^{14}C]$-arachidonic acid. The prostacyclin released from HUVEC was measured as its stable metabolite, 6-keto prostaglandin $F_1\alpha$, using a $[^3H]$ 6-keto prostaglandin $F_1\alpha$ RIA kit (New England Nuclear, Boston, MA, USA).

5)Measurement of ^{45}Ca release from the storage site

We permeabilized HUVEC with saponin by a previously described method[9]. Namely, HUVEC were rinsed with a conditioned buffer solution, buffer B (150mM NaCl, 5mM KCl, 1mM $MgCl_2$, 5mM glucose, 10mM HEPES, 0.1mM EGTA, 0.1% bovine serum albumin, pH 7.4). The cells were incubated for 5 min at 37 °C with 30.0nM Ca^{++}-EGTA buffer solution containing $50 \mu g/ml$ saponin, 140mM KCl, 12mM $NaHCO_3$, 5mM HEPES, 0.42mM NaH_2PO_4, 1mM $MgCl_2$, 5.5mM glucose, 0.1% bovine serum albumin, 5mM creatine phosphate, 10U creatine phosphokinase, 1mM EGTA, and 3.3×10^{-4} $CaCl_2$. After the addition of 1.85×10^5 Bq/ml $^{45}Ca^{++}$(7.1484×10^8 Bq/mg $CaCl_2$, New England Nuclear, Boston, MA, USA), 5.0mM phosphocreatine (PC), 10.0U/ml creatine phosphokinase (CPK), 5.0mM succinic acid disodium salt (Suc), 3.0mM adenosine 5'-triphosphate magnesium salt (ATP), the cells were incubated for 60 min. They were resuspended in 30.0nM Ca^{++}-EGTA buffer solution containing 0.5mM PC, 10.0U/ml CPK, 5.0mM Suc, and 3.0mM ATP after centrifugation at 1500G for 10 min. They were then divided into several tubes (2×10^5 cell/200 μl). After the addition of agents, $200 \mu l$ of cell suspension was dripped on the filter (Whatman glass microfiber filter, GF/C) at every given time interval and vacuumed using a diaphragm vacuum pump (DA-30D, ULVAC Shinku-kikosha, Osaka, Japan) and 1225 Sampling Manifold (Millipore, Bedford, MA, USA) with 30ml of a wash buffer (120mM KCl, 5mM NaCl, 5mM Glucose, 10mM HEPES, 1mM $MgCl_2$, 1mg/ml bovine serum albumin, 1mM EGTA, pH 6.8~7.4). The radioactivity of HUVEC on the vacuum pump filter was measured as residual ^{45}Ca in the cells using a liquid scintillation counter. Residual ^{45}Ca in the cells fell to minimum levels at 10 sec after incubation and following plateau. We calculated the Ca^{++} release by the agents from the storage site for 10 sec as a ratio with the Ca^{++} release by Ca^{++} ionophore A23187.

6) Statistical analysis

Data (expressed as mean ± SEM) were compared using analysis of variance. For F-ratios significant at the 5% level or less, Duncan's multiple range test was applied to determine differences between any two groups. Differences at the 5% level or less (p< 0.05) were considered statistically significant. Percent changes, for which a normal distribution cannot be assumed, were compared using the Kruskal-Wallis non-parametric method for analysis of variance. Whenever the chi-square test results were significant, the Mann-Whitney test was used to determine the significance of the differences between pairs of means.

RESULTS

1) Change in cytosolic Ca^{++} concentration

In the resting state, when the extracellular Ca^{++} was chelated with EGTA, $[Ca^{++}]i$ decreased in HUVEC. The addition of A23187($10^{-6}M$) or $CaCl_2$(1.8mM) to resting HUVEC increased $[Ca^{++}]i$. However, pretreatment with 1mM EGTA inhibited this increase (Fig.1). The addition of thrombin remarkably increased $[Ca^{++}]i$. The stimulation induced by thrombin was reduced by pretreatment with EGTA. Although pretreatment with the protein kinase-C inhibitor H-7 did not reduce $[Ca^{++}]i$ in resting cells, the thrombin stimulated-increase of $[Ca^{++}]i$ was slightly reduced by H-7 (Fig.2).

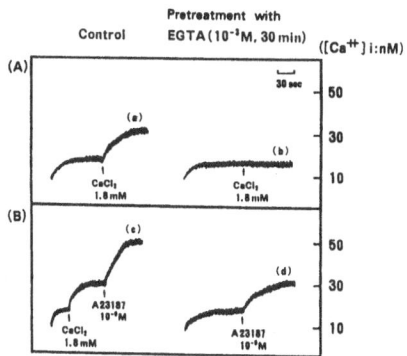

Figure 1 :
Effects of pretreatment with EGTA (10^{-3} M) on the cytosolic free Ca^{+} concentration of human umbilical vein endothelial cells.

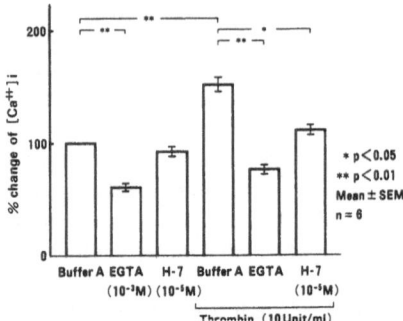

Figure 2 :

Effects of thrombin (10 Unit/ml) on the cytosolic free Ca$^+$ concentration of human
umbilical vein endothelial cells ; Effects of pretreatment with EGTA (10^{-3}M) or H-
7 (10^{-5}M) on the thrombin-induced increase in free Ca$^+$ cocentration of human
umbilical vein endothelial cells. Data are expressed as mean ± SEM (n = 6 ;
*,** represent P<0.05, P<0.01 respectively).

2) PGI$_2$ generation

The addition of buffer A increased PGI$_2$ generation in a time dependent
manner. This increase reached a plateau at 15 min. Pretreatment with EGTA or
H-7 did not inhibit this basal PGI$_2$ generation. The generation of PGI$_2$ from
HUVEC was enhanced by thrombin in a dose-dependent manner. When HUVEC were
pretreated with EGTA or H-7, the thrombin-induced enhancement of PGI$_2$
generation was reduced (Fig.3).

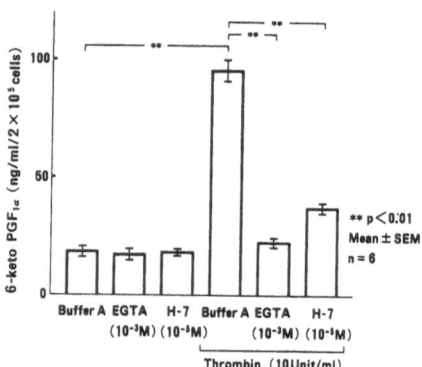

Figure 3 :

Effects of pretreatment with EGTA (10^{-3}M) or H-7 (10^{-5}M) in the resting or
thrombin-stimulated PGI$_2$ generation by human umbilical vein endothelial cells. Data
are expressed as mean ± SEM (n = 6 ; ** represents P<0.01).

3) Effects on intracellular pH

After the addition of 1.8mM CaCl$_2$, [pH]i was slightly alkalized. When
extracellular Ca^{++} was chelated with EGTA, [pH]i was slightly acidified. The
addition of thrombin caused a biphasic shift in [pH]i. Initially there was a brief
acidification of [pH]i. This was followed by a rapid alkaline shift. In cells

pretreated with EGTA, the initial decrease in [pH]i was abolished and subsequent alkalinization was inhibited. The C-kinase inhibitor H-7 inhibited thrombin-stimulated alkalinization, although H-7 did not change [pH]i in the resting state (Fig.4).

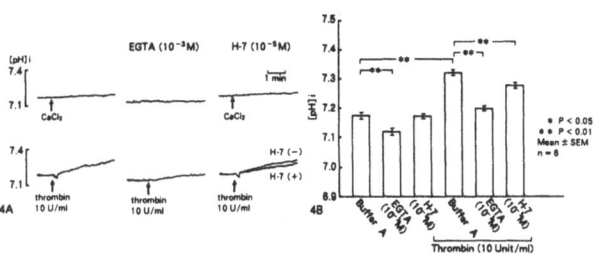

Figure 4A, 4B : Effects of thrombin (10 Unit/ml) with or without pretreatment with EGTA (10⁻³M) or H-7 (10⁻⁵M) on the intracellular pH of human umbilical vein endothelial cells. Data are expressed as mean ± SEM (n = 6 ; *,** represent P<0.05, P<0.01, respectively).

4) ^{45}Ca release from the storage site

IP₃ increased Ca⁺⁺ release from storage sites in saponin-treated HUVEC. This increase was 35.7% of the increase caused by A23187. Pretreatment with 10^{-5}M antimycin or 5×10^{-6}M oligomycin did not inhibit the increase caused by IP₃. This result suggested that IP₃ increased Ca⁺⁺ release from the non-mitochondrial Ca⁺⁺ pool. When cells were alkalized to a [pH]i between 6.8 and 7.4, the Ca⁺⁺ release by IP₃ depended on the alkalinization of [pH]i (Fig.5).

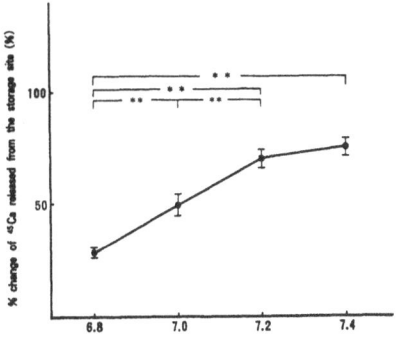

Figure 5 :
Effects of the intracellular pH on the release of ^{45}Ca from storage sites by IP₃ of human umbilical vein endothelial cells. Data are expressed as mean ± SEM (n = 6 ; *,** represent P < 0.05, P < 0.01, respectively).

Discussion

Vascular endothelial cells have recently been shown to display an antithrombotic action via the generation of PGI$_2$[10], tissue plasminogen activator[11], or thrombomodulin[12]. PGI$_2$ effectively inhibits platelet secretion and aggregation. PGI$_2$ inhibits platelet aggregation by stimulating adenylate cyclase, leading to an increase in cAMP levels in the platelets. The regulation of PGI$_2$ generation depends on the activation of phospholipase A$_2$. Recent findings indicate that bradykinin, thrombin, or ATP activate phospholipase C and elevate $[Ca^{++}]_i$ via phosphatidyl inositol turnover. This increase of $[Ca^{++}]_i$ may activate phospholipase A$_2$[13]. Crutchley et al[14] reported that the calmodulin inhibitor W-7 reduces the activation of phospholipase A$_2$. This result suggests that calmodulin contributes to the activation of phospholipase A$_2$. In addition, the activation of protein kinase C contributes to PGI$_2$ generation[15]. In this study, we investigated the effects of $[pH]_i$ on PGI$_2$ generation by vascular endothelial cells because the relationship between $[pH]_i$ and PGI$_2$ had not been investigated.

A rise in $[Ca^{++}]_i$ in the resting state or an increase induced by thrombin causes alkalinization in HUVEC. In contrast, when extracellular Ca^{++} was chelated with EGTA, $[pH]_i$ was slightly acidified and the alkalization induced by thrombin was decreased. The protein kinase-C inhibitor H-7 inhibited thrombin-stimulated alkalization, although H-7 did not change $[pH]_i$ in the resting state. These results suggest that $[pH]_i$ is partly dependent on the extracellular Ca^{++} of HUVEC not only in the resting state but also during thrombin stimulation. On the other hand, $[pH]_i$ is not dependent on protein kinase C in the resting state, but the alkalization of $[pH]_i$ is dependent on the activation of protein kinase C when HUVEC are stimulated by thrombin. In many cells, it has been shown that a rise in $[Ca^{++}]_i$ and the activation of protein kinase C may activate Na^+/H^+ exchangers and alkalize $[pH]_i$[16,7]. However, the mechanisms for the regulation and activation of the Na^+/H^+ exchanger have not been completely elucidated.

Thrombin induces the alkalization of $[pH]_i$ and an increase in PGI$_2$ generation. In HUVEC pretreated with EGTA, the above-mentioned alkalization and increase were inhibited. The protein kinase C inhibitor H-7 diminished thrombin-induced alkalization and increases in PGI$_2$ generation. This result demonstrates that not only an influx of extracellular Ca^{++} but also protein kinase C contributes to thrombin-induced alkalization and increases in PGI$_2$ generation.

Our previous data showed that IP$_3$ enhances the release of Ca^{++} from storage sites in HUVEC. In the present study, IP$_3$-induced release of Ca^{++} from storage sites was enhanced concomitantly with the alkalization of $[pH]_i$. This result suggests that the alkalization of $[pH]_i$ contributes to the antithrombogenic effects of vascular endothelial cells by the increasing PGI$_2$ generation through a rise in $[Ca^{++}]_i$ via increased release from Ca^{++} storage sites.

Acknowledgments

This work was partly supported by Grant-in-Aid for Scientific Research (C)

No. 02807090 and Grant-in-Aid for the Encouragement of Young Scientists No.03770500 from the Ministry of Education, Science and Culture of Japan.

References

1)Molski TFP, Naccache PH, Volpi M, Wolpert LM, and Sha'afi RI. (1980) Specific modulation of the intracellular pH of rabbit neutrophils by chemotactic factors. Biochem Biophys Res Commun 94:508-514

2)Segal AW, Geisow M, Garcia R, Harper A, and Miller R. (1981) The respiratory burst of phagocytic cells is associated with a rise in vacuolar pH. Nature 290:406-409

3)Simchowitz L. (1985) Intracellular pH modulates the generation of superoxide radicals by human neutophils. J Clin Invest 76:1079-1089

4)Royal DS, Yvonne WB, and George HD. (1989) Role of Intracellluar pH in the Axolemma and Myelin Induced Proliferation of Schwann Cells. J Neurochem 52:1576-1581

5)Toyoda T, Sawada S, Niwa I, Maebo N, Tsuji H, Mikami K, Rin K, Nakagawa M, (1985) Effect of Ca antagonists on PGI_2 generation in cultured human vascular endothelial cells; relationship between intra-and extracellular Ca^{++} and cyclic nucleotides. Blood & Vessel 16:245-257

6)Grynkiewicz G, Poenie M, Tsien RY, (1985) A new generation of Ca^{++} indicator with greatly improved fluorescence properties. J Biol Chem 260:3440-3450

7)Rink TJ, Tsien RY, and Pozzan T, (1982) Cytoplasmic pH and free Mg^{2+} in lymphocytes. J Cell Biol 95:189-196

8)Thomas JA, Buchsbaum RN, Zimniak A, and Racker E, (1979) Intracellular pH measurements in Ehrlich asites tumor cells utilizing spectroscopic probes generated in situ. Biochemistry 18:2210-2218

9)Burgess GM, McKinney JS, Fabiato A, Leslie BA, and Putney JWJr. (1983) Calcium pools in saponin-permeabilized guinea pig hepatocytes. J Biol Chem 258:15336-15345

10)Moncada S, Gryglewski R, Bunting S, Vane JR, (1976) An enzyme isolated from arteries transforming prostaglandin endoperoxides to an unstable substance that inhibit platalet aggregation. Nature 263:663-665

11)Levin EG, Marzec U, Underson J, Harker LA, (1984) Thrombin stimulates tissue plasminogen activator release from cultured human endothelial cells. J Clin Invest 74:1988-1995

12)Maruyama I, Salem HH, Majerus PH, (1984) Coagulation factor Va binds to human umbilical vein endothelial cells and accelerates protein C activation. J Clin Invest 74:224-230

13)Hallam TJ, Pearson JD, and Needham LA, (1988) Thrombin-stimulated elevation of human endothelial-cell cytoplasmic free calcium concentration causes prostacyclin production. Biochem J 251:243

14)Crutchley D.J.,Ryan J.W.,Ryan U.S., Fisher G.H., (1983) Bradykinin-induced release of prostacyclin and thromboxanes from bovine pulmonary artery endothelial cells. Biochem.Biophys.Acta 751,99

15)Demolle D, Boeynaems JM, (1988) Role of protein kinase-C in the control of vascular prostacyclin:study of phorbol esters effect in bovine aortic endothelium and smooth muscle. Prostaglandins 35:243

16)Moolenaar WH, Tertoolen LGJ, and de Laat SW, (1984) Phorbol ester and diacylglycerol mimic growth factors in raising cytoplamic pH. Nature 312:371-374

17)Mix LL, Dinerstein RJ, and Villereal ML, (1984) Mitogens and melittin stimulate an increase in intrcellular free calcium concentration in human fibroblasts. Biochem Biophys Res Commun 119:69-75

IS PLATELET CYTOSOLIC FREE CALCIUM AND SEROTONIN CONCENTRATION AND BLOOD VISCOSITY DIFFERENT BETWEEN HYPERTENSIVE AND NORMOTENSIVE SUBJECTS?

Yu-An Ding, Tz-Chong Chou, Ronald Huan

Department of Medicine, Tri-Service General Hospital, National Defense Medical Center, Taipei, Taiwan, Republic of China

Yu-An Ding, M.D., PhD, FRCP, FACC, Department of Medicine, Tri-Service General Hospital, No.8, Sec.3, Ting-Chow Rd. Taipei, Taiwan, R.O.C. FAX: 886-2-3652379, TEL: 886-2-3683028

INTRODUCTION:
The ability of cells in the vascular wall as well as platelets in calcium handling plays an important role in the pathogenesis of certain cardiovascular diseases and is found to be defective in hypertensive states. It is known that calcium plays a central role in the mediation of platelet function and maintenance of blood pressure. Serotonin (5-HT), a highly vasoactive amine, is another factor that has numerous vascular effects. Abnormalities of platelet 5-HT contents and kinetics may therefore affect vascular reactivity and platelet function as well . Since blood viscosity is a determinant of total peripheral resistance, which in turn is an important factor in the determination of arterial pressure, therefore changes in blood viscosity and other rheologic parameters are also seen in hyper-tensives or peripheral vascular diseases. In this study, we want to compare the difference in platelet intracellular calcium, serotonin concentration, and blood viscosity in normotensives and hypertensives.

MATERIALS AND METHODS
Subjects: There were 65 hypertensive volunteers entered in the study with their age ranging from 50 to 69 years with a mean average of 57.7 ± 2.0 years of age. Average mean height and weight are 160.8 ± 2.2 cm and 67.4 ± 1.2 kg respectively. There was no distinction between male and female subjects. These patients were diagnosed to have essential hypertension but were free from any systemic or mental illnesses. All were untreated and ensured to be free from any other medications at least 2 weeks before the study started . Healthy normotensive controls number 25, has an average age of 53.7 ± 1.7, height of 165.6 ± 5.6 cm and weight of 61.2 ± 2.3 kg (Table 1).

METHODS:

1.Platelet calcium concentration
According to the method described by Rink et al,the ACD-anti-coagulated blood was centrifuged for 10 min at 160g to obtain plateletrich-plasma (PRP). The PRP was in cubated with Fura-2-AM $(2.5 \mu M)$ for 40 minutes at $37°C$, and centrifuged, washed and suspended in the above Tyrode's solution.
Platelet number was counted by Coulter counter (model ZM) and adjusted to 2x10 platelets/ml. Basical fluorescence (F) was measured with Jasco CAF - 100 Caanalyzer (Ex= 340nm, Em= 490nm). Maximal fluorescence (Fmax) was gauged after addition of $40 \mu M$ digitonin , minimal fluorescence (Fmin) was measured after addition of 9 mM EGTA.
2.platelet serotonin concentration determination
According to the method of Honegger et al, PRP is centrifuged to 10000g for 5 minutes and the platelet pellet is sonicated in 1ml (50g trichloroacetic acid, 0.5g EDTA, 10 mg sodium matabisulfite).

The sample is left in ice for 5 min, then centrifuged at 10000g for 5 min. Twenty ml of the supernatant fluid is injected into the fluid chromatography with electrochemical detection to calculate the serotonin concentraion.

3.Whole blood and plasma viscosity determination

A 5 ml of venous blood was placed in a plastic tube containing 7 .5u / ml sodium heparin. The whole blood viscosity was measured within 30 min at five dfferent shear rates (212, 106, 42, 21,5 sec) with a Wells - Brookfield viscometer and plasma viscosity were measured at 106 sec. Each blood sample was determined in duplicates and all reading were obtained with reference to standard oil. All measurements were performed at 37℃.

4.Red cell deformability measurement

Red cell deformability is measured as blood viscosity at high shear rate divided by plasma viscosity (high value indicate low deformability).

5.Red-cell flexibility (RCF) determination

Red-cell flexibility was measured by the centrifugation technique .Briefly, capillary whole blood microhematocrit tubes are centrifuged at 200g for 2 minutes precisely. The RCF is expressed as the initial packing rate per min.

RESULTS

The hypertensive (HT) group had a significantly higher blood pressure (BP) level of 147 ± 6/102 ± 3 mmHg. When compared to the normal control (NT; BP: 124 ± 8/79 ± 5 mmHg, p< 0.01, Table 1) with a mean arterial pressure (MAP) of 119 ± 4 mmHg, the HT group had a total plasma calcium (mg/dl) of 9.3 ± 0.21, platelet intracellulr calcium (Ca)of 165.4 ± 12.6 nm and a platelet serotonin value of 0.28 ± 0.03 / 10 platelets. This, in comparison to the NT group, having an MAP of 94 ± 5 mmHg, plasma calcium of 9.2 ± 0.22 mg/dl , Platelet calcium of 118.9 ± 12.4 nm (p<0.05, when compared to the HT group) platelet serotonin of 0.38 ± 0.03 nmol/10 platelets (p<0.05), the refore statistically significant (Table 2).

The hematocrit of the HT group ws 45.3 ± 1.1 and this was signifi-cantly higher than 41.4 ± 0.9 of the NT group. Whole blood viscosity (CPS) at shear rate (sec) of 212 was 4.31 ± 0.09 (HT), 3.89 ± 0.11 (NT), (P<0.05); at shear rate of 106 , 4.68 ± 0.11 (HT), 4.54 ± 0.10(NT); at shear rate of 42, 5.35 ± 0.1(HT), 5.37 ± 0.14 (NT); at shear rate of 21, 6.26 ± 0.13 (HT), 6.25 ± 0.18(NT); at shear rate of 5, 9.66 ± 0.31(HT); 9.61 ± 0.29(NT); at shear rate of 1, 28.3 ± 0.08(HT); 25.6 ± 1.0(NT);(P<0.05) Table 3 and 4.

If hematocr it was adjusted to 45%, at shear rate of 212, whole blood viscosity was 4.21 ± 0.25(HT); 3.96 ± 0.9(NT); at shear rate of 106, 4.40 ± 0.09(HT); 4.33 ± 0.12(NT); at shear rate of 42, 5.19 ± 0.12(HT); 5.02 ± 0.14(NT); of shear rate of 21, 6.20 ± 0.15(HT); 5.82 ± 0.15(NT); at shear rate of 5, 9.78 ± 0.30(HT), 8.71 ± 0.31 (NT) (P< 0.05); at shear rate of 1, 25.6 ± 1.1(HT); 21.0 ± 1.3(NT) (P<0.05). Plasma viscosity in the HT group (1.62 ± 0.05) was significantly higher than the NT group (1.45 ± 0.24) (p<0.01) (Table 3,4).

Plasma fibrinogen was 268.8 ± 7.5 mg/dl in the HT group while the NT group has a value of 240.3 ± 12.7mg/l (p<0.05). Red cell flexibility (RCF) was 19.6 ± 0.43(HT) and 15.4 ± 0.6(NT)(P<0.01) RCF 40 was 21.8 ± 0.4(HT), 20.2 ± 0.43(NT)(P<0.05) RBC deformability was 2.82 ± 0.04 in the HT group and was 3.09 ± 0.11 in the NT group (p<0.05) Table 5.

DISCUSSION:

In previous studies, some have found values of platelet

intracellular calcium concentration exhibited overlap between hypertensives and normotensives, although there were other groups that found elevated basal platelet intracellular calcium concentration in hypertension. This may suggest that there may be other factors as ide from platelet calcium handling that affects BP, such as serotonin and blood viscosity. In our study, our results showed that platelet in tracellular calcium was indeed significantly higher in the HT group (p<0.05). This is in agreement with the findings of Duggan et al claiming that platelet intracellular calcium is elevated in young hypertensives, irregardless of age. Although the mechanism of action responsible for the elevation of platelet intracellular calcium concentration in hypertension is not fully understood, there is however evidence for a relationship between elevated platelet intracellular calcium concentration and platelet aggregability as seen in patients with thromboembolic disorders. Therefore, normotensives with age - related rise in platelet intracellular calcium concentration also has increased platelet reactivity and thereby tempting us to believe· this is due to the elevated calcium concentration in platelets. Also, age - related changes in platelet intracellular calcium concentration in the elderly hypertensives was increased antihypertensive response to treatment with calcium antagonists. Since there is no change or difference in plasma calcium concentration between the NT and HT groups, we therefore assume that it is the platelet cytosolic calcium concentration that is responsible for hypertension and its cardiovascular consequences.

Many studies have shown ketanserin, a selective S2 serotoninergic antagonist, to be effective in blocking the hypertensive effcts of serotonin (5-HT). Other studies have linked 5-HT2 receptor-mediated mechanisms in thromboembolic complications seen in hypertensives. A decrease in platelet 5-HT has been described in hypetension due to release of 5-HT from activated platelets. In our study, we have shown significantly lower platelet serotonin (p<0.05) in our HT group , thereby confirming this fact.

Arterial pressure is dependent on cardiac output andtotal peripheral resistance. The latter is in turn determined by the caliber of resistance vessels and the intrinsic viscous resistance to blood flow ,. Thus, blood viscosity is a determinant of total peripheral resistance.

Past reports have shown abnormally increased blood viscosity in hypertensive patients. Later, more studies evaluated on the rheologic basis for the increase in blood viscosity, namely, the hematocrit, red cell aggregation, plasma viscosity, and fibrinogen, levels which were all elevated in hypertensives. In our study, blood viscosity at a high shear rate of 212 sec was significantly higher in hypertensive than the normal controls. We would be tempted to attribute this for the high hematocrit levels in hypertensives but when the hematocrit was adjusted to 45% , blood viscosity in hypertensives was significantly higher at a low shear rate of 5 sec and 1 sec- which may imply that other factors aside from the hematocrit were reponsible for the elevated blood viscosity such as increased fibrinogen levels and red cell aggregaion. Indeed , we can see from Tabel 5 that all the other parameters such as fibrinogen , red cell flexibility, and RBC deformablity were all higher in the HT group. With higher blood viscosities, prognosis is related to the development of cardiovascular diseases as in angina pectoris , acute myocardial infarction, and peripheral vascular disease. Another therapeutic consideration is in treatment of hypertension; drugs that reduced blood viscosities may be favored over those that increase blood viscosity such as diuretics.

In summary, we have shown that higher platelet cytosolic calcium concentration, whole blood viscosity and plasma viscosity were noted in hypertensives which may in turn be due to the increase in

hematocrit, plasma fibrinogen, red cell flexibility and deformability
in the HT group. Inversely , plasma 5-HT was much lower in hypertensives suggesting its role in hypertension.

REFERENCES
1. Quan CY : Disfunction of calcium handling by smooth muscle in
   hypertension. Can J Physiol Pharmacol 1985. 63: 366-374.
2. Bohr DF, Webb CR : Vascular smooth muscle membrane in hypertension.
   Annu Ret Pharmacol Toxicol 1988. 28 : 389 -409.
3. Rasmussen H : The calcium second messenger system (two parts). N
   Engl J Med 1986. 314:1164-1170.
4. Vanhoutte PM. Luescher TF. Serotonin and the blood vessel wall J
   Hypertens 1986; 4(suppl 1) : S29-S35.
5. Van Nueten JM. Vanhoutte PM. Serotonin and vascular function . Clin
   Anaesthesiol 1984 ; 2: 363-382.
6. Chien S: Blood rheology in hypertension and cardiovascular disease
   . Cardiovasc Med 1977; 2:356-360.
7. Tibblin C. Bergentz SE, Bjure J. et al. : Hematocrit, plasma protein
   . plasma volume, and viscosity in early hypertensive disease. Am
   Heart J 1966; 72:165-176.
8. Letcher RL. Chien S. Laragh JH : Changes in blood viscosity accom-
   panying the response to prazosin in patients with essential hypertension. J Cardiovasc Pharmacol 1979; 1 (suppl): 8-20.
9. Rink TJ, Smith SW., Tsien RY. Cytoplasmic free calcium in human
   platelets : Ca thresholds and Ca-independent activation for shape-
   change and secretion. FEBS Lett 1982; 148: 21-26.
10. Honegger CG, Burri R, Lungemann H. : Determination of neurotrans-
    mitter systems in human cerebrospinal fluid and rat nervous
    tissue by high - performance liquid chromatography with on-line data
    evaluation. J Chromatog,1934, 309, 53-61.
11. Nicolaides AN, Bowers R, Horbourne T, Kidner PM: Blood viscosity
    , red cell flexibility, hematocrit and plasma fibrinogen in patients
    with angina , Lancet 1977; 5: 943-945.
12. Lechi C. Sinigagua D. Corsato M. Covi G, Arosio E. Iechi A Intrace-
    lular free Ca in platelets of essential hypertensive patients.
    Lack of correlation with clinical and laboratory data. J Hum an
    Hypertens 1988. 2:49-52.
13. Astaire C. Levenson J. Simon A. Meyer P. Devynck MA: Platelet
    cytosolic proton and free calcium concentrations in essential hyper-
    tension. J Hypertens 1989. 7:485-491.
14. Lenz T, Haller H Ledersdorg M. Kribben A. Thirde M. Distler A, et al
    : Free intracellular calcium in essential hypertension effects
    of nifedipine and captopril. J Hypertens 1985. 3 (suppl 3) : S13
    -S15.
15. Duggem J, Kiljeatner S, Shericlan J, et al : The Effects of age on
    Platelet intracellular free calcium concentration in normotensives
    and hypertensives. J Hypertens 1991, 9:845-850.
16. Jy W. Ann YS. Shanbaky N, Fernandez LF. Harrington WJ Haynes DH
    : Abnormal calcium handling by platelets in thrombotic disorders.
    Circ Res 1987, 60:346-355.
17. Buhler FR. Kiowski W: Age and antihypertensive responseto calcium
    antagonists. J Hypertens 1987., 5 (Suppl 4): S111-S114 .
18. Janssen PAJ : Pharmacology of potent and selective S2-serotonergic
    antagonists. J Cardiovasc Pharmacol 1985; 7 (suppl 7) : S2-S11.
19. Fetkovska N, Amstein R, Pletscher A, Buhler FR : Impact of age,
    gender and hypertension on serotonin -dependent platelet function
    (Abstract). 12th Scientific Meeting of the International Society
    of Hypertension, Kyoto, 1988.

20. Amstein R. Fetkovska N, Luscher TF, Kiowski W, Buhler FR: Age and the platelet serotonin vasoconstrictor axis in essential hypertension. J Cardiovasc Pharmacol 19888, 11 (suppl 1) : S35-S40.

21. Guciheney P, Baudouin -Legros IM. Valtier D. Meyer P: Reduced serotonin content and uptake in platelets from patients with essential hypertension: is a ouabain -like factor involved? Thromb Res 1987, 45:289-297. 22.Palermo A, Bertalero P. Pizza N. Merati MG, Borchini M, Libretti A : Enhanced platelets serotonin release after adrenergic stress in arterial hypertension. J Hypertens 1987, 5 (suppl 2) : S141-S143.

23. Guyton AC :Arterial pressure and hypertension . Circulatory Physiology. III Philadelphia W.B. Saunders Co. 1980.10-29.

24. Schloz PM, Karis JH, Gump JM, et al. Correlation of blood rheology with vascular resistance in critically ill patients. J Appl Physiol 1975,39 : 1008 - 1011.

25. Chien S, Usami S, Dellenback RJ, et al: Comparative hemorheology. Hematological implictions of species differences in blood viscosity. Biorheology 1971; 8:35-57.

26. Kannel WB, Gordon T. Wolf PA, et al. : Hemoglobin and the risk of cerebral infarction : the Framingham Study, Stroke 1972; 3: 409-420.

27. Chien S, Usami S, Dellenback RJ, et al.: Shear-dependent interaction of plasma proteins with erythrocytes in blood rheology. Am J Physiol 1970 : 219 : 143 - 153.

28. Letcher RL, Chien S, Pickering TG, et al. : Direct Relationship between blood pressure and blood viscosity in normal and hypertensive subjects. Am J Med 1981 ; 70: 1195-1202.

Table 1

Comparison of Blood Pressure in Normotensive (NT) and Hypertensives (HT)

	n	Age (years)	Height (cm)	Weight (Kg)	SBP (mmHg)	DBP (mmHg)
NT	25	53.7 ± 1.7	165.6 ± 5.6	61.2 ± 2.3	124 ± 8	79 ± 5
					**	**	**
HT	65	57.7 ± 2.0	160.8 ± 2.2	67.4 ± 1.2	147 ± 6	102 ± 3

** P< 0.01

Table 2

Comparison of Blood Pressure, Intracellular Calcium and Serotonin Concentration in Normotensive (NT) and Hypertensives (HT)

	n	MAP (mmHg)	Plasma Calcium (mg/dl)	Platelet (Ca 2+) I (nmol/ l)	Platelet Serotonin (nmol/ 10^8 platelet)
NT	25	94 ± 5	9.2 ± 0.27	118.9 ± 12.4	0.38 ± 0.03
				*	*
HT	65	119 ± 4	9.3 ± 0.21	165.4 ± 12.6	0.28 ± 0.03

* P< 0.05

Table 3
Comparison of Hematocrit and Blood Viscosity in
Normotensives (NT) and Hypertensives (HT) Patients

| | | | Whole Blood Viscosity (CPS) | | |
| | | Hematocrit | shear rate (sec^{-1}) | | |
	n	(%)	212	106	42
NT	25	41.4 ± 0.9	3.89 ± 0.11	4.54 ± 0.10	5.37 ± 0.14
HT	65	45.3 ± 1.1 *	4.31 ± 0.09 *	4.66 ± 0.11	5.35 ± 0.11
		adjust hematocrit to 45%			
NT			3.96 ± 0.09	4.33 ± 0.12	5.02 ± 0.14
HT			4.21 ± 0.21	4.40 ± 0.09	5.19 ± 0.12

* $P < 0.05$

Table 4
Comparison of Hematocrit and Blood Viscosity in
Normotensives (NT) and Hypertensives (HT) Patients(cont'd)

| | | Whole Blood Viscosity (CPS) | | | |
| | | shear rate (sec^{-1}) | | | Plasma |
	n	21	5	1	Viscosity
NT	25	6.25 ± 0.18	9.61 ± 0.29	25.6 ± 1.0	1.45 ± 0.24
HT	65	6.26 ± 0.13	9.66 ± 0.31	28.3 ± 0.8	1.62 ± 0.05 * **
		adjust hematocrit to 45%			
NT		5.82 ± 0.15	8.71 ± 0.31	21.0 ± 1.3	
HT		6.20 ± 0.15	9.78 ± 0.30 *	25.6 ± 1.1 *	

* $P < 0.05$; ** $P < 0.01$

Table 5

Comparison of Plasma Fibrinogen, Red Cell Flexibility (RCF)
and Deformability in Normotensives (NT) and Hypertensives (HT)

Variable	NT	HT
Fibrinogen (mg / dl)	240.3 ± 12.7	268.8 ± 7.5 *
RCF	15.4 ± 0.6	19.6 ± 0.43 **
RCF40	20.2 ± 0.43	21.8 ± 0.4 *
RBC deformability	3.09 ± 0.11	2.82 ± 0.04 *

* $P < 0.05$; ** $P < 0.01$